FELDENKRAIS METHOD:
TEACHING BY HANDLING

Keats Titles of Related Interest

THE FELDENKRAIS METHOD: TEACHING BY HANDLING

A Technique for Individuals

YOCHANAN RYWERANT

Illustrations by Daniela Mohor

Keats Publishing, Inc. New Canaan, Connecticut

THE FELDENKRAIS METHOD: TEACHING BY HANDLING

This book is published in association with the K. S. Giniger Company, Inc., Publishers, 250 West 57th Street, New York, New York 10107.

Designer: Jim Mennick

Library of Congress Cataloging-in-Publication Data

Rywerant, Yochanan
    THE FELDENKRAIS METHOD
    Bibliography: p.
      1. Manipulation (Therapeutics).   2. Sensory-motor integration.
  3. Self-perception.   4. Feldenkrais, Moshe, 1904–1985.   I. Title.
RMII724.R97   1983   6L6.7'40622   83-47734
ISBN 0-87983-544-0

Printed in the United States of America

Published by Keats Publishing, Inc.
27 Pine Street (Box 876)
New Canaan, Connecticut 06840-0876

Contents

Part IV: Working Through Sessions

Part V: Some Illustrative Case Histories

Foreword

Yochanan was a teacher of physics in one of the best schools of Israel. He was at that twenty-eight years running.

Later he joined the Feldenkrais School. He worked thirteen and a half years within close quarters in the same room in which I worked. He has his own "handwriting" like all the others. Everyone learns the method without imitating his teacher. Yochanan is not imitating anybody.

The book in front of you should be reread several times. That way you are likely to get most of the goodness of the book. Good luck!

M. FELDENKRAIS
Tel Aviv, Israel

Preface

The Feldenkrais Method: Teaching by Handling is a momentous publication, because it makes accessible a unique form of human education. The book is a presentation of the system of Functional Integration devised by the Israeli scientist Dr. Moshe Feldenkrais. The Feldenkrais system is a way of handling the body by communicating specific sensations to the central nervous system in order to improve the functions of the motor system.

Functional Integration is unique in that it evokes changes in the human brain at a level heretofore thought unachievable by any known educational technique: muscular tonicity—even spasticity—is actually modified, the range of movement is enhanced, movement becomes more coordinated, and the overall efficiency and comfort of muscular functioning is increased.

In *The Feldenkrais Method: Teaching by Handling* Yochanan Rywerant has devised a framework for understanding an immensely subtle and elusive technique for human change. Rywerant has successfully created the archetectonics for understanding a major area of human cybernetic functioning and, in so doing, has effectively established the vocabulary for a new area in the field of nonverbal communication. Feldenkrais, the inventor of this new area of Functional Integration, is also its most brilliant practitioner as well as its most inspirational and intuitive teacher. What Rywerant has accomplished is to have taken this intuitive clarity and worked it into an ingenious intellectual framework that makes sense of the technique's elusive subtleties. He has succeeded in removing the mystery from a method that creates remarkable improvements in the motor system with a remarkable economy of means.

The two major uses of this volume are, first, as a textbook for persons wishing to learn the practice of Functional Integration and, secondly, as an explanation of the cybernetic process involved in changing human movement patterns. It is the latter explanation that makes the learning of the Feldenkrais technique far easier than would otherwise be possible. Rywerant has constructed an explanatory superstructure for the technique that makes it clear that there are levels of human communication and transformation whose existence was scarcely suspected before the appearance of Feldenkrais.

Rywerant's conception of the "manipulon" as a basic unit of nonverbal communication is at the heart of this cybernetic theory. And his discussion of the different types of manipulons gives a comprehensive description of the discrete ways in which "handling" can communicate information to the brain. His discussion of the functions of the brain and the central nervous system are clear and very much to the point, and this clarity allows us to understand how the manipulatory sessions have a certain prescribed form and way of proceeding.

Yochanan Rywerant was born November 7, 1922, in Bucharest, Romania. He lived the bulk of his youth in the city of Cernauti (now part of the Soviet Union) until the Second World War. Although he had studied for eight years as a violinist, when he entered the University of Cernauti in 1939 he chose to study mathematics. However, after one year of university work, the war intervened and Rywerant, a Jew, was shipped off to a forced labor camp.

After his liberation at the end of the war, Rywerant attempted to emigrate to Palestine, which was at that time under British mandate. But before he could reach Palestine he was intercepted by the British navy and interned in Cyprus for a period of six months in 1947. In 1948 he managed to escape from Cyprus and, as a stowaway aboard a British ship, reached the

Holy Land, where he adroitly shimmied down a mooring line and set foot for the first time in his adopted land.

Following service with the Israeli defense forces, Rywerant completed his studies in mathematics and physics at Hebrew University, Jerusalem. In 1952 he accepted a post as physics professor in a secondary school in Givataim, a suburb of Tel Aviv. In that same year he married the distinguished Israeli-born composer Yardena Alotin and the two have continued living in Tel Aviv since that time.

Also in 1952 Rywerant first met Moshe Feldenkrais, who had just begun his famous series of Awareness-Through-Movement exercise classes in Tel Aviv. He attended these classes regularly over the next fifteen years.

When in 1969 Feldenkrais decided to teach his technique of Functional Integration, Yochanan Rywerant was one of the fourteen members of this first training group. The training was completed in 1971 after three years. But even before that time, Feldenkrais invited Rywerant to become his first assistant in the Feldenkrais Institute on Nachmani Street. The offer was accepted, and he has continued to work side by side with Feldenkrais up to the present.

In 1973 Rywerant assisted Feldenkrais in teaching an Awareness-Through-Movement class in Berkeley, California, which was the time I met both men. When, in 1975, Feldenkrais accepted my invitation to offer a Functional Integration training program in San Francisco—the first in the United States—Rywerant served as his assistant. This position as teaching assistant continued into the third training program offered by Feldenkrais in 1980 at Amherst, Massachusetts.

Through his work at the Feldenkrais Institute as well as his own private practice, Yochanan Rywerant has become thoroughly experienced in the theory, practice, and neurophysiological foundations of Functional Integration. Thirty years of acquaintance with Feldenkrais have imbued him with a lucid vision of the precision and care necessary for the successful practice of Functional Integration. It is this same vision that informs the pages of this book and offers the reader an authoritative account of the Feldenkrais system with all of the exactitude and subtlety that Feldenkrais demands.

Rywerant has been previously known to the reading public through his four remarkable case histories, which I had the pleasure of publishing in *Somatics* magazine. These case histories appear as the last four chapters of this volume, and they illustrate fully how deliberate, precise, and effective are the techniques of Functional Integration. The wonderful story of Hanoch's return to the flute displays the "miraculous" quality that so often accompanies the practice of the technique, just as it illustrates amply the ability of the human central nervous system to learn new ways of functioning far beyond what most people believe to be possible.

The Feldenkrais Method: Teaching by Handling is a major work in the field of somatics, namely, the field that sees bodily functions as simultaneously a third-person objective event and a first-person subjective event of awareness. What Feldenkrais has demonstrated and Rywerant has explained is that movement can be employed to transform awareness and that awareness can be employed to transform movement: the third-person and first-person aspects are integral functions of the same somatic system.

Yochanan Rywerant has given us a text that springs high above the crippling bifurcation of body and mind. The unity of body and mind are seen as much more than morally evident; Rywerant shows them to be *scientifically* evident. Functional Integration takes advantage of this self-evident fact about human nature and uses awareness as a somatic function that can help change movement functions, with the end result that the change-of-movement functions also change the nature of awareness. In brief, the human individual can, by this method, be taught continued functional growth and continued personal evolution.

Practitioners of Functional Integration will find that *The Feldenkrais Method: Teaching by Handling* offers them dramatically new vistas for the possibilities of their profession. Scientists and laymen who wish to understand the Feldenkrais system and the reasons for its consistent effectiveness will find in Rywerant's volume an introduction that is as substantial as it is rewarding.

Any important new discovery and understanding is, at first glance, complex and too subtle to grasp. Rywerant has taken the complex and subtle system of Functional Integration and has succeeded in conceptualizing and naming procedures and insights that were originally nonverbal. His concepts and precise terminology have made accessible a nonverbal procedure that is of immense importance, not only because of its direct use for human improvement but for its indirect foreshadowing of the farther reaches of human nature.

THOMAS HANNA, PH.D.

Acknowledgments

It is a great pleasure to express my thanks to Prof. Eleanor Criswell and Dr. Thomas Hanna, whose constant encouragement and essential editorial help were so important for the coming forth of this book. Only friends such as Tom and Eleanor could have spent energy and time in the generous way they did.

Daniela Mohor, the artist, showed much enthusiasm and took great pains in preparing the illustrations.

I am indebted to Flora James-Peli for urging me to bring this book out of its embryonic state.

My wife, Yardena Alotin, was constantly at my side and her technical help was invaluable.

YOCHANAN RYWERANT

The information in this book on the Feldenkrais method is not intended as a source of medical advice. The assessment of symptoms and proper diagnosis and therapy can only be provided by a medically qualified practitioner. Before beginning a program of manipulation, make sure that it is medically appropriate for the recipient.

Introduction

Introducing the subject of this book can best be done by recounting one particular case, not a spectacular one, but one which makes clear the special approach that is going to be outlined in the course of these pages.

A. N., a young woman of twenty-five years of age, came to see me upon the recommendation of a friend. She had suffered pain in her lower back for over two weeks and hoped to receive some relief. She said that the same thing had happened once before, a year ago, but that the pain had ceased after a few days.

Looking at her, I observed a slightly bent posture with a sunken chest. Otherwise she had a tall and slender figure. Her spine, from the neck down to the pelvis, formed one continuous, slightly convex curve.

I asked her to lie down on my work table on the side of her body that felt the more comfortable. My table is actually a wide bench, slightly padded for comfort, and about the height of a chair seat. A. N. chose to lie on her left side. I placed a soft support underneath her head. She curled herself up a little bit, so that the curvature of her spine became even more pronounced.

I wondered whether the very tense muscles of the small of the back, especially on her right side, had their antagonists, i.e., the muscles of the stomach, tensing up as well. I found them quite taut, which meant that extra stress was being put on the tired back muscles. This contracted state of the trunk muscles was neither intentional nor conscious. It therefore made no sense to ask A. N. to stop tensing these muscles. Instead, she had to be shown what she was actually doing and what possible alternatives she might have for doing otherwise.

Among other things I did with A. N. was to bring her pelvis and her chest (on the right side) slightly nearer to each other in a gentle fashion. I held them with my hands in this way for a few seconds, released them, and then repeated this same movement. In fact, I was simply doing what these tense trunk muscles seemed determined to do themselves by their involuntary shortening. In fact, by making this same effort with my hands, I was rendering the effort of these muscles superfluous. My message was: "You can rest now, count on me, I am doing your work for you."

After a little while, I could feel that the message had been received. The contracting muscles gradually lessened their effort to shorten the distance between pelvis and chest, and thus they resisted less than before the lengthening of this distance. A learning process had now begun. A. N. perceived—perhaps not wholly consciously—that there was a possible alternative to what had been happening before.

I then did something which clarified this situation further and helped A. N. to familiarize herself with what was going on in her muscular system. After all, the sensation of having such muscles less tensed might be new and nonhabitual for A. N., at least after having had very different sensations for the past two weeks during which she was in pain. I had to provide her with situations in which this newly learned experience could be applied in various contexts.

I looked for functions and movements in her arm and chest that were related to and dependent upon reduced tension in the trunk muscles, and for similar functions in her leg and pelvis.

I checked A. N.'s right shoulderblade, which was held near the spinal column and drawn slightly upwards. It was difficult to slide it away from this position. This was evidently part of the pattern of the back muscles holding the trunk in a rigid state.

Touching along her spine, I discovered (simultaneously for my-self as well as for A. N.) that the muscle group on the right side of the spinal column was also tense in the thoracic and cervical sections all the way up to the base of the skull.

Among other things, I lifted A. N.'s right arm in front of her face, bringing it above her head. With this particular arm move-ment, which was quite far from the contraction in the small of the back, she allowed her right shoulderblade to slide upward with the lifted arm. I wanted the connection between shoulder and lower back to be clarified, so I gently pulled her arm above her head with one of my hands, while with my other hand I touched the muscles in the small of the back. Thus, she eventu-ally became aware through her sensations that with this move-ment of the arm, the chest moved slightly in relation to the pelvis. Meanwhile, I observed that with every movement there was a straightening out of the spine and even a slight arching of the small of the back.

Having clarified this situation, I could then show her that the position of her head, as she was lying, could be very easily aligned with the already lengthened spine. And when A. N.'s breathing became deeper and steadier, I pointed this out to her to make her aware that another function had improved along with the lessening of tension in the trunk muscles.

I put one of my hands on her pelvis and the other on her ribs (still on the right side) and made gentle twisting movements, bringing the chest forward and the pelvis backward, and vice versa. Since I did this in an easy and comfortable manner, with-out provoking any possible feeling of danger, A. N. allowed this without the least resistance.

I now checked the movability of her pelvis, this time manipu-lating her legs, since we are more aware of the movements of the limbs than of the pelvis. A. N. was lying on her back with the legs extended. I raised one of her legs slightly by lifting the heel up from the table three or four inches. I then oriented this leg so that it pointed toward her head, and then I pushed the leg toward her head by pressing the sole of her foot. Making a few small and gentle movements like this, to and fro, the pelvis began to rock easily in a rolling movement. This showed A. N. a way of adjusting the degree of her muscular tonus for easier movements of the trunk.

Something else that became clear to A. N. was that force can easily pass through the skeletal structure without having to involve any muscular effort. The pressure through the legs went all the way up to her head, reminding A. N. of what it felt like to use skeletal support efficiently in an upright position.

Gradually A. N. realized (at least on a sensory level) that if she could become loose and ready for movement and action in any direction without preliminary preparation, then the muscle spasm in the small of her back would be terminated.

With A. N. still lying on her back, I again checked the ease of the movement of both her arms and her head.

A. N. stood up, straightened herself out—her shoulders broad, her chest up—and walked with ease. Her pain had almost completely disappeared.

This is a fragmentary description of a session of Functional Integration. The emphasis was, as the reader could tell, on the motor functions and on the amount of control a person has over these functions. The general principles and some of the technical aspects of this method are the subject of this book.

This system is a way of teaching people to increase both their physical and mental awareness in order to maximize their inherent potential. The human brain, far from being utilized to its full capacity, is capable of some surprising kinds of learning. By being taught to differentiate and combine patterns of action, a person's efficiency, comfort, and well-being can be increased. The person in fact learns how to learn. And someone who develops a conscious attitude towards these possibilities is able to program and reprogram his actions according to changing circumstances. This helps him solve his problems with greater ease.

There are two techniques within this system:

1. group lessons, called Awareness-Through-Movement ses-

sions, during which the teacher advises *verbally* how to do certain movements, which sensations to pay attention to, and how to achieve improved motor functioning, widened self-awareness, and a more adequate self-image;*

2. an individual, manipulatory technique called Functional Integration, through which the teacher can, by gently manipulating the pupil's body, become aware of the peculiarities of the pupil's neuro-motor functioning. Through proper manipulation, he makes the pupil aware of these peculiarities, along with *alternative* ways of controlling the motor functions. The effect of these lessons is very often spectacular, ranging from an improvement in well-being and vitality, and ease and efficiency of motor functioning in general, to a gradual alleviation of pain and a decrease in motor impairment.

Among those who can profit from help of this kind are people who need improved body coordination and people with sensory-motor deficiencies of any kind produced by trauma, disease, or deterioration in structure or function.

This volume deals exclusively with the manipulative technique, Functional Integration. The book will be of relevance to those interested in the problem of increasing efficiency by better coordination, to those who deal with this problem professionally, such as physical educators, dancers, actors, athletes, music teachers, and also medical and para-medical people and psychologists. The book can equally serve as supplementary didactic material for participants in professional courses in Functional Integration. We will not deal thoroughly with the scientific basis of the system, nor will the book provide all of the knowledge of anatomy that is required. For this, the reader must consult the standard textbooks on anatomy, physiology, or neuro-physiology. After working through the book, the reader will still be a beginner, in need of expanding his abilities by sharing experience with senior practitioners of the method.

Moshe Feldenkrais, born 1904, Doctor in Physics, and Direc-

* Moshe Feldenkrais, *Awareness through Movement* (New York: Harper & Row, 1972).

tor of the Feldenkrais Institute in Tel Aviv, devised this general system of neuro-motor teaching and reconditioning. His major theoretical work, *Body and Mature Behavior,* appeared in 1949. After that, he taught both the group and individual techniques, lecturing and teaching professional courses in Israel, the United States, Canada, and many European countries.

Moshe Feldenkrais died in Tel Aviv on July 1, 1985.

Part I

MANIPULATION AND TEACHING

1. Manipulation as Nonverbal Communication Between Teacher and Pupil

One has the ability to control one's actions more or less consciously. Controlling an action means, of course, checking or monitoring one's ongoing activity and correcting, changing, or sometimes stopping its course, according to circumstances. We are self-correcting or self-governing organisms—expressed in modern parlance, *cybernetic entities*. This term summarizes a quite complex state of affairs. Human functioning, as seen from this viewpoint (we will deal here mainly with neuro-motor functioning), can be said to have certain formal characteristics:

1. Not all conceivable occurrences have the same chance or probability of actually happening. Any activity consisting of randomly happening events is governed by the law of equal probabilities, but here randomness is *excluded* by restrictions, limitations, or *restraints* governing the organism's actions. These restraints both diminish considerably the probability of many events happening and heighten the probability of others. Any fairly coordinated movement could serve as an example of an activity subjected to restraints. My writing with a pen, at the present moment, is kept from becoming a meaningless scribble by definite restraints brought to bear on the movements of my

hand.* Restraints of this kind are of several different categories. One category stems from the structure of the organism, bones, joints,' and ligaments and their respective ranges of movement. Others seem to be determined by nerve impulses coming from the central nervous system (CNS), which bring about specific *neuro-muscular patterns*. Initially, it should be remarked that efferent nerve impulses can be part of conscious (deliberate) patterns, of instinctive (inherited) patterns, of learned and then more or less automatically performed patterns, and of patterns conditioned or influenced by various acute or chronic illnesses.

2. An efferent nerve impulse serving to correct or to change any ongoing activity is in most instances elicited by information coming by afferent nerve impulses originating in the sense organs. This is the well-known concept of *sensory feedback*. When it works satisfactorily, the information about any deviations of the motor performance from a preselected course of action will elicit efferent nerve impulses, bringing about a diminution of that deviation (negative feedback). Thus we have a "closed loop" of information flow, and any change anywhere in that loop is apt to elicit changes in the other parts of that loop. The information coming by way of sensory feedback is the source of such "restraints."

It is instructive, for example, to see what happens if you start to write a sentence, then close your eyes and continue writing to the end of the line, without the visual feedback. The ensuing deviations will prove how necessary this feedback is for preventing "disorder." An interesting trait of sensory feedback is *redundancy*. Information received by feedback or otherwise usually exceeds what is really necessary, in the sense that the information could be stripped of many details and still retain its meaning for the recipient: a bad telephone connection might

---

* A good presentation of the basic concepts of bio-cybernetics can be found in Gregory Bateson's *Steps to an Ecology of Mind* (New York: Ballantine, 1975) in the chapter "Cybernetic Explanation" and the following, pp. 399 ff.

still allow a meaningful conversation. Returning to the illustration of writing without visual feedback, if you don't close your eyes but someone merely dims the light in the room, your writing can continue fairly undisturbed. Examples like these show that if information is supposed to transmit patterns, then redundancy is very welcome and must not be considered superfluous. It is essential for insuring the pattern-recognition of the information by the recipient; in other words, it is *essential for communication,* be it sensory feedback or communication between individuals.

3. If we take a closer look at the concept of *pattern of action,* or specifically *neuro-motor pattern,* then cybernetic and system-theoretical considerations will lead us to include in the pattern a little more than the immediate agents engaged, say, in the performance of the movement, which are the sensorimotor cortex, outgoing and incoming neural circuits, and the respective parts of the motor apparatus, muscles, bones, and joints. Actually, all agents interconnected by *information flow* or by *energy* exchange* in the context of the pattern, before or during its performance, should be considered parts of that pattern. In the example of writing, we can consider, of course, the different modalities of feedback: tactile, visual, kinesthetic. I feel the pen between my fingers and adjust the pressure of holding it, I control the pressure of the pen's tip on the paper and the movements of the pen, I control the size of the letters according to what I see, I move my eyes and head in order to follow with my vision the tip of the pen, and so on.

4. Characteristically, feedback is elicited by information coming *with the action* or a short while *after* the completion of some phase of it. Moreover, there is information leading to control of action coming *ahead* of the action (feedforward). This information can be of two kinds. One kind indicates the

---

* "Energy" will be used here and throughout in the *physical* sense.

goal of the action and stems probably from the supplementary motor area of the brain's cortex (the programming "agent").* For example, starting to write a word, I already know the rest of the letters (or even the word's written visual image as a whole), and sometimes many of the words that follow. Another kind of beforehand information leading to control of action stems from the immediate environment and/or parts of my body relevant to the activity. When I see myself gradually approaching with the pen the margin of the sheet, I already anticipate the program for moving over to start the next line. Similarly, if the text to be written is being dictated to me, the auditory input and the parts of the brain dealing with hearing- and speech-understanding provide the "feedforward," ahead of the action itself. We shouldn't underestimate the role of the *environment* as an agent connected by information flow (or sometimes also by energy exchange) with the part of the system involved in a pattern of action. Think, for example, how the pattern of writing changes when I want to jot down a word so that people present will not notice it, or if I have to be careful while writing not to touch or to push someone who sits very near.

5. There is still another cybernetic characteristic to be clarified pertaining to intentional action. "Controlling" my action means also that I can "follow with my attention" the ongoing process (and I am probably doing it most of the time). This monitoring or checking is a prerogative of what we usually call "the conscious mind."** But we should ask: checking against what? A simple introspection will provide the answer: We have "in our mind" a representation or an image (A) of what is going to happen. We get also a picture or an image (B) of what is

---

* For a vivid, experimentally obtained description of the areas of the human cerebral cortex simultaneously involved in different sensory, motor, and mental activities, see Niels A. Lassen, David H. Ingvar, and Erik Skinhoj, "Brain Function and Blood Flow," *Scientific American*, October 1978, pp. 50–59.

** I should explain these quotation marks: these expressions are taken from everyday language, and I hesitate to take them as scientifically well-defined terms.

already happening, and are able to compare both. We can decide eventually to change the course of action or sometimes to change the goal-image. Since these images are built of elements from the various sensory modalities, we could, roughly speaking, consider such checking as a higher level of feedback, but it is more than that. The image B is obtained by integrating a complex amount of sensory information and by *recognizing an emerging pattern*. Then comes the *juxtaposition* of A and B and the decision whether B compares satisfactorily with A or not, followed in the latter case by a change of action, or eventually by a reprogramming of A into some A'.

In our conscious mind we don't think all these processes in words, but rather in a *"language of images."* These images and their different alternatives emerge or recede, are remembered or forgotten, preferred or discarded, loved or feared. This nonverbal language of images and the functions of pattern-discrimination and monitoring is the vehicle through which learning-teaching by manipulation takes place.

6. The images of action-patterns most probably have a neurophysiological counterpart (engrams). How these engrams are encoded and what that code-language might be is still a matter of conjecture. The encoded patterns, whether in the language of engrams or in the language of images, relate to their counterparts in reality as *maps* relate to the *territory* they depict, and so in analogy with other cybernetic systems, we can in *code-language* weigh and compare possibilities, make judgments and decisions, and create new patterns of action, and then we can by action transfer patterns from the "map" into the "territory"—we can execute or perform the pattern. The monitoring of the action, the control of the outcome, is again, after due encoding, done in the map-language.

This complex function of self-governing undergirds the adaptability of the individual and the continuous adjustment to circumstances or to changing goals. Patterns of action are tried out, perfected, and learned. Moreover, the individual also learns about the way to relate, for example, to a *class of patterns*. One learns to learn.*

This learning process starts with birth and goes on during the individual's life, growing in complexity and refinement. With many this growth process stops at a certain stage, or, if conditioned by adverse occurrences in the individual's personal history, even regresses to an earlier stage of development. If one agent (in the sense used before) engaged in a class of patterns has gone wrong, or if one informational pathway between agents is impaired in its function, it can be enough to produce a significant deterioration in the person's way of functioning.

Typically, a trained person can, just by gently touching or moving parts of the involved person's body, get some detailed information about the peculiarities of that person's neuromotor functioning. Moreover, that trained person (whom we shall henceforth call "the teacher") might succeed, by these manipulations, in conveying to the other person ("the pupil") this same information about his own peculiarities. When the pupil appreciates the situation adequately, it becomes possible to be aware of and explore, under the teacher's guidance, alternative ways of functioning and to envisage the changing of patterns that had seemed unalterable. This two-way communication between pupil and teacher travels through the same information-flow channels and involves the same agents engaged in any pattern of action, as I mentioned earlier. But the ensuing patterns of teacher-pupil interaction are more complex, in the sense that they encompass both systems with their respective multimodal sensory links (tactile, kinesthetic, and visual). Such an interaction usually acquires still another dimension or modality: that of empathy. This happens when the pupil feels that the teacher understands the problem and has the intention and ability to help resolve it.

At an initial stage, the teacher might become aware of the pupil's *impaired ability to change patterns of movement*, or

---

* Gregory Bateson called this learning of a higher logical type "deuterolearning." (See *Steps to an Ecology of Mind*, pp. 166 ff.)

even to "passively" allow such a change. The "restraints" (structural and functional, subsistent or transitory) come into the awareness of both teacher and pupil. In a further stage the pupil's ability to discern small differences between patterns is enhanced. That ability to judge small differences in sensory input is obviously essential in making any attempt to reprogram patterns of action.

Usually one finds that unsatisfactory functioning carries with it an inadequate or *incongruent representation* of patterns of action as images in the pupil's conscious mind. Not only can the "wrong" thing be felt to be "right" and vice versa, but the image of what is being done differs, sometimes strikingly, from the action actually done. A quite simple example should suffice to explain what is meant by incongruity of representation. It is a common practice to raise a cup to the lips while lifting the elbow, so that hand and arm, up to the shoulder, are moving as one rigid piece. One might *not be aware* that one is acting differently from someone who leaves the elbow still and slightly pronates the forearm together with an appropriate extension of the wrist. The cup is being taken to the lips in both cases, and the elbow and its place in space is not part of the image representing the action; hence the representation is incongruent. It is not contended that any of the two possible patterns (and there are more, of course) are not legitimate, if acted out deliberately. But the superfluous, unnecessary activation of the bigger (proximal) muscles around the shoulder joint and the scapula produce a movement which lacks the efficiency, the ease, the elegance, and even the satisfaction that goes with a refined movement done with the smaller (distal) muscles of the forearm and the hand. Moreover, the fixing of the elbow joint and wrist joint might turn out to be habitual (not under control) and therefore a hindrance to any more refined and skilled task.

The teacher will have to provide the pupil with the opportunity to *experience* and *compare* other possible patterns. It is like "updating the maps" of patterns in the language of images and making them more adequate to the pupil's actual actions. Good mapping abilities are needed for planning ahead, as with voluntary actions, where the image of what is going to be carried out —the "blueprint map"—precedes the action itself.

It should be remembered that such a way of enriching the repertoire of patterns by trying out, experiencing, and comparing different possibilities—and all that *playfully*—is just the way every human being learns most of the voluntary actions *from earliest childhood:* coordinated and differentiated movement in the field of gravity, reactions to sensory stimuli (proprioceptive, environmental, social), communication, speech (the mother tongue), and the like. This way of playing-learning is thus known in everyone's experience, and is felt to be familiar. Judged by its results, it can be considered a most efficient way of learning, and so this process of learning should be mimicked in the teacher's work. The style of the manipulatory technique will be set in accordance with these insights.

The *strategy* of this manipulatory teaching technique entails establishing for the pupil efficient ways of self-direction by helping to reprogram the pattern of action towards increased adaptability. But then the *tactics* consist in setting up situations that give the pupil the possibility to start playing-exploring, trying out new options, or remembering old forgotten ones. These are the *learning situations* that the teacher will have to create. As for the pupil, a feeling of security, of not being endangered by what is going to happen, and a comfortable ambience will allow the *natural curiosity* to come into play. Proposed new patterns should never startle the pupil but rather emerge easily, out of secure patterns established earlier in life or even reflex reactions of the neuro-motor system (the stretch reflex, righting reflexes, and others). The only things that should be allowed to "come as a surprise" to the pupil are the insights about how the system has been functioning until now and what better alternatives there are.

As with any communication system, so it is with our complex system of pupil-teacher-environment: we have to deal mainly with sequences of stimulus and response, rather than cause and effect.* This is related to the fact that any self-governing biological system has its own energy source acting collaterally to the pathways of information; in other words, the energy that is used for the response flows in a different channel than the energy that provides the stimulus. For example, if the doorbell rings and I stand up and walk over to answer it, then I am using my own energy for that. It is not the impact of sound waves on my tympana that brings me physically to my feet. Conversely, if someone else uses force and carries me to the door, this could hardly be considered interaction by communication. The two channels are related in the sense that a flow of information through the sensory channel (the stimulus) might, so to speak, trigger a flow of energy through the motor system, as part of the response. Such a relationship between two channels, where a change in the flow in the one brings about a change in the other, is called a *relay*.

This is also the case with the stimulus-response interaction. The *energy of the response* is usually *provided by the respondent*. On the other hand, the *energy exchange* that comes with the reception of the stimulus might be quantitatively *insignificant*, although the *information* content might be *considerable*.

The knowledge we have about sensory perception and about the way nerve impulses travel indicates that a sensory neural impulse is triggered by a change in a stimulus, a *difference*. The unchanging stimulus is without information content.

Even a slow and continuous increase or decrease in stimulus might not be perceived as such. A step-like change in the stimulus will start an afferent nerve impulse that carries information. Differences in stimuli are subject to the Weber-Fechner law in physiology: The least perceptible difference in stimulus is a definite fraction of the stimulus already present. If the least perceptible difference of a stimulus S is designated by $\triangle S$,

---

* Ibid., p. 403.

then: $\frac{\Delta s}{s} = k$. The law holds relatively true for stimuli of medium strength, which is the relevant situation in this context. The actual value of the constant k is different for the different sensory modalities. For example, for the sensation of pressure (as in supporting a weight), it is 1/40. This means that only a change of weight greater than 1/40 of the weight originally supported will be perceived. Differently put, in order to be able to perceive very small differences in stimuli, the overall excitation must be brought down.

It follows from the foregoing that there are ample reasons for concluding that an effective, communicative manipulation should result from a quite small energy exchange. It should then have a chance of creating a learning situation, where playing-exploring is feasible, where no danger is anticipated, where refined differentiations are possible, and thus where a partial reprogramming can take place.

The more the energy exchange in a manipulatory interaction is limited, the greater is the information content that has a chance of being transmitted. In other words, the active part of the manipulation being small, the sensory information flow between teacher and pupil (in both directions) can go unhindered. Conversely, a forcefully done manipulation will on the one hand blur the teacher's ability to evaluate the desirable limits of the actions, and on the other hand it will put the pupil on the defensive—obviously not conducive to a learning situation—where what is being done to him will at best be tolerated.

It is possible to summarize the foregoing in a quasi-mathematical way. If I postulate (somewhat arbitrarily) that the two quantities in question (the energy exchange $\triangle E$ and the information exchange $\triangle I$ in a manipulatory interaction) are inversely proportional or that their product is constant—which is saying the same—then I can write:

$$\triangle E \cdot \triangle I = K$$

an equation that could be represented graphically by a hyperbola. Actually, K sets an upper limit to what could be attained

Fig. 1. Energy Exchange and Learning

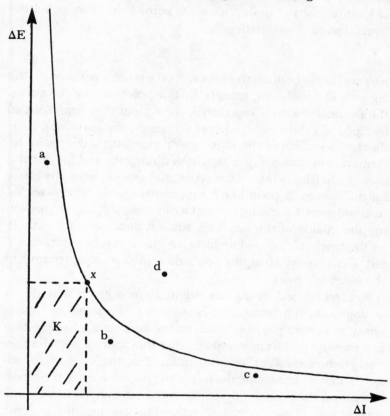

ΔE: energy exchanged
ΔI: information transmitted
 a: violent manipulation
 b: fairly good manipulation
 c: good learning by efficient manipulation
 d: situation incompatible with this style of manipulation

in any short manipulatory sequence. We have to add the sign of inequality, because the product can also be less than K, as in the case of an inefficient manipulation done with a certain energy exchange, and the useful information resulting from it being less than maximal. The product could even be zero, when at least one of the multiplicands is zero. K may be called the "quantum of manipulation."

$$\Delta E \cdot \Delta I \leqq K$$

Any rectangle built on the axes and on a point x situated on the curve is of equal area, namely K. For points below the curve, the respective area is less than K. Any point may represent an instance of a short manipulatory sequence, the horizontal coordinate (the width of the rectangle) representing the useful information exchanged (perhaps both directions) and the vertical coordinate (the height of the rectangle) representing the transmitted energy. A point like b represents a fairly good teaching manipulation. Changing to point a, for example, means worsening the quality of the teaching, since it denotes much activity on the teacher's part, while little information is being transmitted. Conversely, changing towards c means improvement in the teacher's work.

Readers versed in physics might have noticed that this is analogous to the formula of Heisenberg's Principle of Uncertainty in atomic physics, which states, concerning the position of a particle and its momentum, that they cannot both be precisely determined at the same instant. The smaller the imprecision in determining one, the larger the imprecision in the other. Moreover, the product of both imprecisions can never be made smaller than Planck's constant, named the "quantum of action." Here, of course, the inequality sign appears reversed for the reason that K is postulated to set an upper limit to the product of variables involved, whereas in particle physics there is a lower limit for imprecision in determining the two quantities involved.

2. The Approach to Communicative Manipulation

In order to be able to use the foregoing ideas and principles, the teacher has to be oriented almost continuously to the pupil's own world of perceptions, feelings, and images. The teacher should be, during the manipulative session, a part of the pupil's environment. Setting up a learning situation means first of all to free the pupil, as far as possible, from the usual preoccupations and from any worry about what is going to happen next. Kinesthetically, this means it is necessary to adjust the body to the demands placed by the gravitational field on the pupil's movements, muscular tonus, and posture. These demands are usually met by habitual, stereotyped patterns, and an effective way of temporarily neutralizing these patterns is to have the pupil lie down on a horizontal surface (a couch or a table), in reasonable comfort.* A supine or a prone position might be appropriate, and if in some instances it is felt (by the teacher or by the pupil) that this is not secure or quiet enough, then the pupil may lie on one side, knees drawn up, with some soft support put underneath the head (the fetal position).

With the proprioceptive and exteroceptive stimuli changed and the general muscular tonus perhaps lessened, the pupil will be able to appreciate any information coming through the teacher's handling in a context different from the habitual, es-

---

* For a thorough explanation of this point, see Moshe Feldenkrais, *Body and Mature Behavior* (New York: International Universities Press, 1950), p. 120.

pecially if the teacher succeeds in devising situations and complex movements that are felt as "new" and "different," though being done in a most gentle way. The pupil will then recognize the manipulations as being mainly *informative* and not *formative;* in other words, providing information and not trying to bring about change. Sometimes special *meta-communicative signals* are called for to make this distinction clear to the pupil. These are messages *about* the kind of communication intended to take place. It can happen, for instance, that the pupil will interpret, on a more or less conscious level, a certain movement done by the teacher as a cue to initiate a habitual movement pattern, instead of merely experiencing the new information that comes with that handling. The teacher could then stop, for example, and after a while start a similar manipulation again, but with a much smaller amount of movement. The pupil might then come to recognize the discrepancy between this very small stimulus and the habitual, disproportionate response. With this insight the pupil can begin to interpret the incoming information differently, and is able then to halt his stereotypical reaction and learn a different one. Sometimes there may be the need for a verbal remark as a meta-communicative message, but even then, the sensory discrimination remains the decisive event.

More than one level of control in the pupil's system might be involved in clarifications of this kind. As is known, there are several *hierarchical levels of control* of neuro-motor functioning in the CNS, the lowest being the level of spinal reflexes, and the highest, the level of conscious, deliberate actions. Actions learned long ago and now quite automatically performed are on some intermediate level. However, the effector system, including lower motoneurons, peripheral nerves, and skeletal muscles, is the *same one* for all levels, and it so happens that any hierarchical level of control subordinates and inhibits by its very action the lower levels and so diminishes the likelihood of movement patterns typical of some lower level to arise.

Something like this will take place when I decide, for example, to breathe or to walk "differently" for a little while, perhaps changing the rhythm or the pace, or deliberately adding elements of movement that are not part of the "automatically" emerging pattern. The teacher might sense the operative level of control in the pupil's CNS revealed in the pupil's response to any pattern tried out with manipulative interactions; and, in case such a pattern is eventually changed, the level of control will be raised, at least temporarily, with the teacher's help. This help consists in *supplying necessary ingredients* of a different pattern of action, which will either replace the previous pattern or enable the pupil to choose the new and different pattern.

Although such a process of creating new patterns for the pupil is for the teacher mostly a nonverbal sequence of images, movement, sensory perceptions, and the like, the teacher should nevertheless be able to describe *verbally* (at least to himself) the pupil's functioning as it reveals itself, as well as the manipulative interaction as it unfolds. It is true, of course, that a description of any neuro-motor process can be carried out on *several descriptive levels*, each one presenting a different aspect of an inherently complex occurrence. To avoid confusion, it is a good idea to differentiate the levels of description initially. Here are some of the more commonly used *levels of description* for neuro-motor processes. The levels mentioned are not exhaustive, and the designations are mainly for identification.

1. *The kinesiological level:* Movements are described in terms of the skeleton, joints, muscles, acting forces (gravity, muscular forces, frictional forces, elastic forces, inertial forces), momentum of moving parts, and the like, using mechanical models and abstractions such as levers, balance, stability, and rigidity.

2. *The representational level:* Action is described in terms of the image of that action in the individual's mind (these images constituting the map-language) and the changes in the performance of an action (changes in the "territory") produced by

changes in the corresponding image, as well as the changes in the image produced by changes in the action.

3. *The functional level:* At this level of description any action is seen as the carrying out of some biological function (including what are considered higher intellectual functions). A biological function can be any of the following: breathing, eating, walking, gaining stability in the gravitational field, seeking comfort, defense against danger (real or anticipated), aggression, orientation in the immediate environment, communication, any intimate behavior, and so on. Questions about the interdependence of body structure and function, about efficiency or economy in energy expense, about any kind of learning, improvement or deterioration of a function, and about the level of consciousness on which a function is carried out can be expressed and approached at this level of description.

4. *The cybernetic level:* This is the level of description on which the first half of chapter 1 is laid out. Information is flowing between different parts of the CNS, the body, and the relevant parts of the environment, these parts (or agents) relaying, processing, storing, or originating information. Most of the non trivial activity is, or seems to be, goal-directed, and the interaction of the different agents achieves control or self-direction towards attaining the respective goal. That control is possible on several levels, which constitute a hierarchical buildup of "superior" levels controlling their "inferiors."

It is possible to make a graphic display of certain classes of activities by drawing up "information-flow maps," on which the different agents are represented by squares ("black boxes") connected with lines representing the channels of information flow. Some of these symbols might easily be correlated to the respective anatomical or physiological items, some with more difficulty. We might, for example, know quite well the nature of the nervous impulse as a vehicle of information, but the nature of the agents having to do with memory (information storage) or pattern recognition has still to be elucidated, although functions like the above-mentioned are obviously involved. Following the symbols used by Prof. D. M. MacKay,* I shall illustrate this approach by presenting a tentative information-flow map for the *manipulative interaction of teacher and pupil* (fig. 2). Two stages are envisaged. The first stage relates to the situation in which the teacher does some manipulation, such as exploring the pupil's habitual ways of responding, and the pupil responds in his habitual way. The second stage relates to a changed response of the pupil, following a possible clarification or insight.

In face of the incompleteness of this picture and of the fact that some of the functions still await more elucidation by neurophysiological research, I choose not to deal with the correlation of the pictured agents and the respective parts of the CNS.

The basic feedback loops for both the teacher and the pupil are depicted. The field of interaction is where the actual manipulation is carried out (the teacher's hand and the touched or moved parts of the pupil's body), as well as where the sensors are located that produce the related afferent impulses of both the teacher and the pupil. The teacher's effector system *(E)* carries out the activity chosen by the selecting agent *(S)*. Sensory information is gathered by the sensory integrator *I* and evaluated by agent *V*. Here this information is compared with the goal of the action indicated by the Programmer *(P)* and any mismatch is fed back to the Selector *S*, which changes the activity accordingly. This closes the basic feedback loop. Some sensory information might directly affect the selection independently of the indicated goal. This is the feedforward *(ff)* elucidated in chapter 1.

With the teacher there is additionally a higher-order loop. The sensory information gathered by *I* enables him to discriminate a certain pattern in the pupil's response (agent *pd*) and the Programmer *(P)*, working in close collaboration with Memory

---

* D. M. MacKay, "Cerebral Organization and the Conscious Control of Action," in *Brain and Conscious Experience,* ed. J. C. Eccles (New York: Springer-Verlag, 1966), pp. 422–45.

Fig. 2. Information Flow Map for Non-verbal
Communicative Manipulation

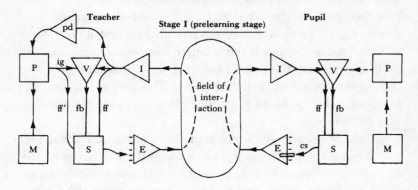

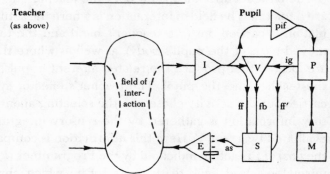

I: integrator of sensory information (indicates state of affairs)
V: evaluator of the mismatch of the state of affairs and some goal
    or habit
S: selection of form of activity
E: effector with range of activities
pd: pattern discriminator
P: programmer
M: memory
ig: indication of goal
fb: feedback
ff: feedforward
ff':   higher-order feedforward
pif: pattern image formation or recognition
cs: compulsive selection
as: alternative selection

(M) (whether short-term or long-term), preselects the activity by a higher-order feedforward *(ff')*.

In Stage I, the pupil's basic feedback loop works the same way, except that the selection of the activity is possibly made "compulsive" by a predetermined, habitual way of acting *(cs)*.

In Stage II, the learning stage, the pupil recognizes the emerging image of a possibly new pattern. Agent *pif* uses this information coming from *I* and passes the result on to *P*. A higher order feedforward loop is thus created and the selection done by *S*, which now gets the additional input *ff'*, might no longer be compulsive *(as)*.

5. *The neuro-physiological level:* The parts of the nervous system and notably the various parts of the brain are considered in terms of their functions, connections, and localization. The nervous impulses flowing and connecting different locations in the nervous system constitute the activity of the system.

One of the standard ways in neurophysiology of determining the functions of various anatomical parts of the brain is, for example, to correlate brain injuries or other lesions at definite anatomical locations with specific functional impairments.

Research in this vast area is going on continuously, and new methods of investigation are being devised.

6. *The neuronal level:* This is a refinement of the former level. Individual cells in the brain cortex have been explored, for example, by stimulating them electrically (through microelectrodes) and recording the response of the individual, or by recording the cell's electrical activity (again through microelectrodes) during certain peripheral stimulations or activities. By other methods, the connections between individual neurons have been studied. Gradually some understanding of the functions of certain cell groups and cell layers is emerging.*

---

* The lay reader is referred to the September 1979 issue of *Scientific American;* all the articles in the issue deal with different aspects of brain physiology. The last two levels of description are treated there, but also the chemical level and, to a lesser extent, the cybernetic level.

All of these levels of describing neuromotor activity are of course legitimate—each of them emphasizing a different aspect of that activity. The *complete* picture, however, is a synthesis of at least several levels of description. Many a controversy in these matters could be spared simply by a consensus concerning the exact level of description involved and its appropriate concepts and assumptions. Even the classical controversy of mind versus body seems often to be only a failure to recognize two concepts as being two levels of description of the same complex phenomenon.

I would suggest that the reader be attentive to the different levels of description as they are used in the following text, since transitions from one level to the other will have to occur for the sake of expediency. The three levels mentioned first (the kinesiological, the representational, and the functional) will be used primarily, but an understanding of the cybernetic and neurophysiological levels is also desirable.

Part II

THE BASIC
TECHNIQUE

3. The Unit of Communicative Manipulation (The Manipulon)

The prospective teacher of Functional Integration will have to be especially sensitive to the pupil-teacher relationship in three areas: *findings* in relation to the pupil, the *actions* that the teacher might initiate, and the pupil's *responses* to the situation. This kind of "calibration" of the teacher's senses can be attained gradually by trying out various manipulations in variable situations and with different persons assuming the role of the pupil. These should be tried out first, and then, at a later stage, combined into more meaningful sequences. Since any manipulation should relate to the three above-mentioned areas, even the smallest bits of communicative manipulation will have to be conceived accordingly. For the purpose of conciseness I shall call these small manipulative units *manipulons.**

"Manipulon" will henceforth be the term used for any short manipulative sequence having as constituents: (*a*) some preliminary knowledge or information about the structure and the functions involved (some of a general character, but some necessarily related to the pupil), (*b*) the action proper (the teacher "proposing" to the pupil certain changes through manipulation, and (*c*) the pupil's response or reaction to these manipulations as perceived by both the teacher and the pupil

---

* I have coined the word "manipulon" in analogy with terms used in particle physics, such as proton, neutron, electron, photon, and so on. Some of these particles are said to be "exchanged" between interacting particles.

(thus creating additional information). Manipulons will, in the following pages, be described so that they can be practiced by the reader. The active phase will of course be the easiest to describe in words or pictures. Concerning the preliminary information and the pupil's response, these will gradually become distinctly definable, while the reader accumulates experiences that will reveal the manifold variety of body structures and possible ways of reacting. Manipulons will also be *repeatable units,* repeated not merely for the reader's benefit but also primarily in actual teaching—to render a certain situation clearer to the pupil or to help the pupil become familiar with it.

If, during the repetitions of any manipulon, new information surfaces or the pupil's response changes (perhaps after a new insight), then the ongoing manipulon will have to be considered a *different manipulon,* obviously having a different relevance in this new context (see, for example, Stage II in figure 2). It follows that different manipulons might have the same active phase and therefore be described visually in the same manner, although they might have different "meanings." For example, a pupil might in the course of similar manipulons think any of the following thoughts: "That's something I have never done before"; "Sure, I remember now, but I have to see how I'll be using that back home"; "That's easy now, but a week ago that movement was still painful"; or "Oh, nothing new in that! Waste of time!"

The manipulons proposed should be tried out at this stage *only* with grownup, healthy, preferably young people serving as "pupils." Friends or members of the family should fill this role at first.

One should make it clear to the "pupil" that there will be some gentle, inoffensive movements, done for the purpose of clarifying to the reader some practical details of the technique, and that they have no therapeutic purpose. *The pupil is ex-*

pected to allow these movements, if possible, without helping or resisting.

Most manipulons are done with the pupil lying in a specified position *on a padded bench* or table, approximately 42 cm. (17 inches) high, while the teacher stands or sits in an appropriate place nearby. A small seat the same height as the bench will usually serve the purpose best.

Familiarization with the intended style of manipulation will come through a few series of manipulons. These are described for one side of the body only, but should be tried out on both sides, although not necessarily with the same "pupil."

For example, have the pupil lying on his back, legs extended and arms alongside the body, while you are positioned near the right shoulder.

Take the pupil's right arm, the elbow not fully extended, and lift it up so that the humerus comes to be approximately vertical (fig. 3). One good way to grasp the arm in that position (try other ways as well, and then decide which serves the purpose best) is to have the right palm underneath the elbow, the four fingers on the inside, the thumb supporting the elbow from the outside. The left hand takes the wrist, or the forearm very near the wrist, with the palm facing the pupil's right palm. *The grasp should be gentle, with the surface of the hand rather than with the fingertips.* Try now to feel the weight of that arm. If the manner of holding the arm provides a feeling of ease and security, the pupil might eventually cease to support the arm, and you will surely feel the weight of it pressing on your hands. To do this, you may have to extend your own elbows slightly.

Starting from that position it will be easy to produce various *basic movements of the elbow in space.* Note first of all that by moving the entire arm as one piece, for example (in order to do that it is necessary to coordinate the movements of both arms), no movement is made in the elbow joint, and any change of the elbow's position in space (relative to the rest of the pupil's body) may mean movement in the shoulder joint and perhaps the

Fig. 3

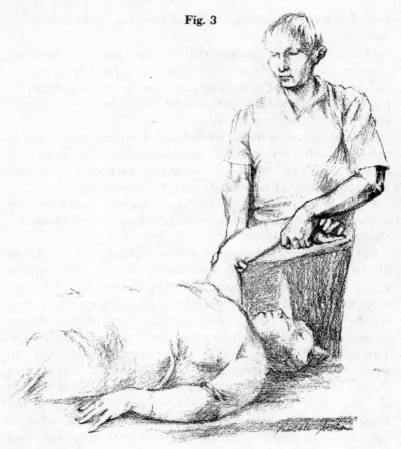

chest as well, and so on. Make a few repeated *small* movements of the arm up and down* (slight extension and flexion in the shoulder joint). These movements should appear as preparatory to "real" movements that might follow, and as if checking for possible resistances. Make the movements slowly, one or two seconds in each direction. Finish by stopping at a point midway

---

* Up, down, right, left, front, and back will be considered throughout *relative to the pupil's frame of reference* unless differently worded. "Up towards the ceiling" means vertically up, but "up" with the pupil supine means toward a horizontal position, in the direction in which the pupil's head is pointing.

between such possible obstacles. Now, make left and right movements, in the same manner as before, with the forearm remaining parallel to the pupil's body (adduction and abduction), and look for a "neutral" position.

There is another way of moving the elbow left and right, namely, by keeping the wrist fixed in space (this adds rotation of the humerus). Take the easier of the two ways first ("easier" means from the pupil's point of view). One may succeed in perceiving *differences in the pupil's ability to allow the movements*. If it happens that this ability changes (improves), it can be considered one's help in bringing the pupil's control—in that context at least—to a higher level. Now isolate the rotation of the humerus around its own axis: having the elbow slightly flexed as before, move the wrist up and down (horizontally), while keeping the elbow's place fixed.

Holding that right arm as before, and nearest to what appears to be a "neutral" position in respect to the different directions, lift it alternately up, away from the pupil, and let it return to the original position, so that the upper arm moves along its longitudinal axis. Start with very small movements.

This manipulon can show to a certain extent the degree of adjustability the pupil has with the functions involving the upper arm and the shoulder blade. After a few trials with different persons on both sides of their bodies, you will probably become aware of an increasing variety of responses. For example, how far is the scapula allowed to move and how easy is the movement? What happens with the chest, the head? The character of the scapula's participation will change sometimes during the repetitions. If not, think about a possible shortcut to achieve this change. Try any of the following and decide which might be more appropriate in each instance: (1) with a very easy grip, hold the pupil's wrist stationary in space somewhere in front of the face with the fingers dangling down, so that by lifting the upper arm, the movement of the *elbow* in space is emphasized; (2) change the grip by holding the pupil's right elbow with the left hand, the forearm resting on your left fore-

arm, and help the lifting with your right hand or fingers underneath the scapula; (3) with the left hand as in (2), assist the
lowering of the scapula (which you might expect otherwise to
occur because of the arm's weight) by pushing slightly on its
outer edge, somewhat below the armpit; (4) add some verbal
remark, such as : "Let me just have your elbow"; or "You seem
to resist me. Let us see if you have to. Resist me now on purpose,
yes! Resist now again, but less than before. Good, now stop
resisting."

Verbal advice should be kept to a minimum, and the reader
will find in due course that he conveys most of the necessary
communication *nonverbally*. Words can be semantically am-
biguous, eliciting different associations for different people.
Some words are emotionally loaded, such as "tension," "stress,"
and "relaxation"; they might therefore detract from the play-
ing-exploring-becoming aware quality of Functional Integration.

Next, have the pupil lying on the back, knees drawn up and
the soles of the feet on the bench, so that the legs are slightly
spread as in standing. Check some of the basic movements of
the knee in space. The joint mainly involved in this is of
course the hip joint. Lift the pupil's right leg so that both the
hip joint and the knee joint are bent at right angles, the lower
leg horizontal. Do this by supporting the ankle with the right
hand (all the fingers on the inside of the ankle), while the left
hand is somewhere on the knee (fig. 4). Feel the weight of the
leg. Remember now to produce the movements in the same
manner as before, starting with very small movements and
watching for any reaction that might point to the pupil's adjustability and the degree of command over that adjustability.
There might be a "neutral" area midway between some possible "obstacles" or between the limits of the range of movement. This neutral area can be used as a starting point for
moving in a new direction. First, move the leg in and out, so
that it remains parallel to its initial position (adduction and
abduction of the thigh). Then move the ankle in and out, the
lower leg still horizontal, while keeping the knee stationary

Fig. 4

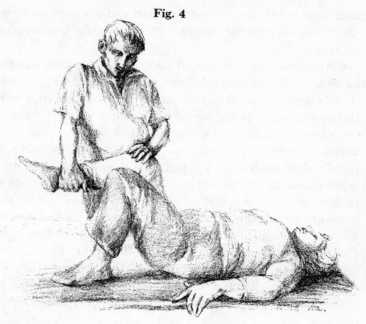

(rotation of the thigh). Now combine both elements, by moving the knee in and out, while the ankle is either held in place or moved in the opposite direction. If the last movement is gently executed, it may be possible with some pupils to detect the limits of rotation in the hip joint as determined by the joint's structure.

It often happens that the situation at the hip joint or around it makes rotation to the limit painful. A great variety of conditions might have this as a symptom. Someone suffering from any of these conditions will usually try to avoid going to the limit, either by stiffening the muscles around the hip joint (thus reducing the range of the thigh's rotation), or by utilizing the pelvis to help turn the knee. The latter saves some of the rotation in the hip joint by having some movements in the lumbar vertebrae instead. The movement of the knee in space is then not reduced, and any irritated site at the hip joint gets its rest at the same time. Without such a condition at the hip joint, any utilization of the pelvis will increase all the more the range of that movement. Consequently, we should consider that second way of coping with the situation a more efficient level of adaptability.

Coming back to this second series of manipulons, you might observe, while rotating the thigh, what happens with the pelvis. If the participation of the pelvis, especially when approaching the movement's limits, seems to you unsatisfactory (and even the mere rotation in the hip joint is felt to be resisted and avoided), then you can try the following: keep on holding the pupil's right ankle with the right hand, and while guiding the ankle outwards (inward rotation of the thigh), help the pelvis by pushing slightly with the left hand from behind the great trochanter towards the pupil's head, so that the leg and the pelvis *move as one unit* (fig. 5). Repeat a few times, without helping the pelvis return to its original position. Produce a similar movement in the opposite direction (outward rotation of the thigh), this time helping the pelvis by a gentle push in the right groin, away from the head. As before, leg and pelvis move as one unit.

Fig. 5

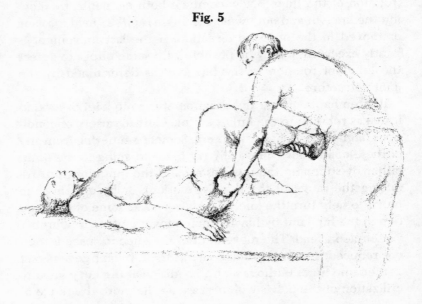

When producing these *nondifferentiated movements*, two things usually occur: The pupil has the feeling of "no movement in the hip joint" and thus becomes able to give up some of the defense patterns around that joint, and secondly, the pupil becomes aware of possible movements of the pelvis connected with movements of the knee in space. By trying the *differentiated movement* again (the rotating of the thigh relative to the pelvis), both you and the pupil will observe the ease and increased range of movement.

Have the pupil lying on the left side, the knees bent and pulled forward comfortably. Put a soft support underneath the head, so that the neck will be aligned comfortably with the dorsal spine.

Check now the movability of the pelvis relative to the chest in the following manner. Stand behind the pupil and find the right pelvic crest (crest of ilium) by easy palpation. With the left hand press gently in the area between the pelvic crest and the great trochanter toward the sternum (fig. 6). If you push gently enough, you will discover the exact direction in which *this* pupil is allowing some easy movement of the pelvis. Press again, but let the pelvis return "by itself" to the original position. Now help with the right hand from behind the great trochanter. Observe that both hands move tangentially to an arc of a circle having its center on the bench, where the pelvis is being supported.

With the hands in the same position, continue to make the movement while gradually changing the emphasis to the "coming back," so that ultimately the pressure will cause the pelvis to roll away from the pupil's face. Observe during this time what happens with the chest, the shoulders, and the head. The pupil will allow them sometimes to roll slightly up and down, simultaneously with the pelvis. Observe the pupil's breathing. When intending to push the pelvis up and seeing the start of a breathing-in movement, wait until the breathing-in is completed, then push, trying to not interfere too much with the rhythm of the breathing.

Fig. 6

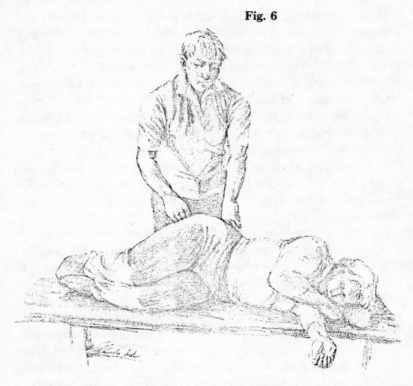

Have the pupil lying supine, arms alongside the body, and sit at the head. Put the right hand, palm down, gently on the pupil's forehead, so that your forearm, wrist, palm, and fingers are all horizontal, parallel to the pupil's shoulder girdle. Keep them horizontal throughout the series. With almost no pressure on the forehead, roll the head slowly to the left and then back to the center. Start with the smallest perceptible movement and keep the force so small that it compares with the force needed to slide the skin of the forehead over the underlying skull. Don't try to find the limits of that movement's range. Rather appreciate the regularity (or irregularity) of the resistance you meet. Coming to an "obstacle," don't try to overrun it by increasing the force. On the contrary, reduce the force, and explore easily the adjacent areas (on either side of the obstacle) for smoothness. Eventually, the character of that spot of resistance might change, usually becoming "smoothed out." Watch for the breathing movements and see whether they relate sometimes to what you are doing. You may use the left hand for the right half of the range.

Have the pupil lying on the stomach, the left ear on the bench, the left arm alongside the body, the right arm bent, so that the palm is lying down somewhere in front of the face, and the right knee drawn up sideways, so that the thigh is at a right angle to the spine. Sit facing that knee and gently roll the right leg towards the pelvis, letting it return to the original position by itself. It is a small but clear movement of the thigh along its own axis. Observe the movement of the pelvis. Is there, in addition to its sideways roll, a component of either flexion or extension? Even if not, you can still do the following: By gently pushing on the appropriate side of the great trochanter simultaneously with the rolling of the leg, you can now slightly exaggerate that additional component, which may seem "parasitic-like" in the sense that it is added without being necessary or increasing efficiency. After a few repetitions, and feeling the movement clearly outlined, change the additional element into its opposite (rearranging the hands accordingly).

Now put the left hand somewhere in the middle of the pupil's spine, the fingers "holding a few vertebrae in place" by their spinal processes, while applying pressure with the right hand, as before, through the knee or the leg (fig. 7). The place on the spine where this can be done efficiently has to be found in each instance. By this manipulon, it becomes clear (to both the teacher and the pupil) that the movement of the knee forward and backward involves a certain bending and twisting of the spine.

This position, as well as the increased movability of the pelvis, can be used as a starting point for another series of manipulons. Slightly push the right side of the pelvis towards the head by applying some pressure from behind the right great trochanter,

Fig. 7

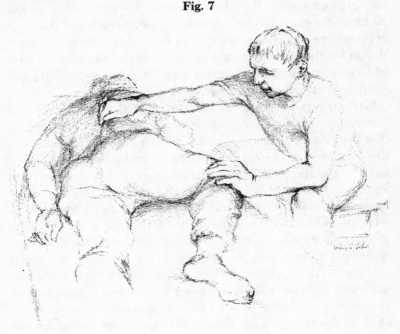

or behind the right ischium (the sitting bone). Release and repeat again. Observe the way the spine participates in this—
perhaps a lateral back-and-forth bending. Observe the movements of the head and the left shoulder. Try also to produce this
movement in a steady rhythm, selecting the timing (the frequency) that yields the easiest response by the smallest force.

See if you can now produce *the same movement* by pushing
the left shoulder in the direction opposite to the one in which
it was moving before, as if with the intention of helping what
was previously the return movement. One way to do that might
be the following: Sit facing the top of the pupil's head, make a
vertical surface out of the fingers of the right hand as they are
bent down at the knuckles, apply the back side of the bent
fingers on the pupil's left shoulder near the neck, and extend
your right arm in a direction that coincides with the direction
of the intended push, that is, towards the pelvis, but slanting

slightly downward (fig. 8). Use the least possible force. Observe whether the pupil's right hip moves away with the pressure, together with an appropriate lateral bending of the spine. Now try a rhythmical movement as before, and after getting the right timing, reach out with the left hand and touch the right pelvic crest, not applying pressure but merely "going with the movement" (the right arm need not be extended). This will increase the likelihood of the pupil becoming aware of the movability of the pelvis and of the way it is connected with the movements of the spine.

Fig. 8

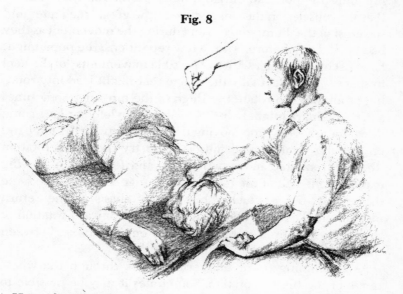

Have the pupil lying on the stomach, the legs extended, the head facing to the right, the right forearm in front of the face, the left arm alongside the body, and the feet slightly apart, say shoulder-wide. Sit facing the pupil's left thigh. With the right hand, support the pupil's left shinbone from underneath, near the ankle, and bring the lower leg into a vertical position. Keep it that way by a very gentle grip. Now tilt the leg slightly *away from you,* so that the thigh rolls on the bench (outward rotation of the thigh), and *come back to the vertical,* while keeping the right angle at the knee unchanged. As with previously described examples, look for the degree of smoothness and regularity with which the pupil is allowing the movement. During the movement it is easy to find with your left hand the great trochanter as it changes its position relative to the pelvis. Follow that movement with the hand. If that movement seems smaller than expected, don't push harder, but make it "easier for the pupil to take" by slightly lifting the pelvis from underneath the anterior superior spine simultaneously with the tilting away of the leg, so that there is barely any movement in the hip joint (the nondifferentiated movement). You may observe that the muscles on the side, between the great trochanter and the crest of the ilium, stop tensing during the movement as they had been doing before. After a few repetitions, the pupil might have become familiar with the possible movements "of the heel in space." This is actually the image that might lead into rotating or allowing to rotate the thigh in the hip joint. Sometimes a verbal remark might help: "Why don't you let your *heel* come down there?" Now stop moving the pelvis, leaving the left hand on the above-mentioned muscles, and try the initial rotation (the differentiated movement) back and forth again. Having explored one half of the movement's range, continue the same movement, but gradually shift the emphasis to the return movement. Then tilt the leg *towards you* (inward rotation of the thigh). This time, put the left hand on the muscles between the trochanter and the sacrum.

As a summing up of this series, check through the whole range of the thigh's rotation. Sometimes it may be possible to detect the limits of the range of movement. Observe how the pelvis is participating at these limits.

Have the pupil lying on the stomach, with the legs extended, the heels turned outward, the head facing to the left, the left forearm in front of the face, and the right arm alongside the body. Place yourself near the pupil's left side, facing the pelvis. Find by easy palpation the left-side arc of the pelvic rim, somewhere below the ribs. Use the concavity of the pelvic bone just below that line and press there slightly, along an imaginary line pointing to the sternum. Use the smallest force possible and feel free enough to alter the direction slightly, if necessary, until the pelvis moves in the easiest way.

Now observe the movement of the spine produced by pushing the pelvis. It is probably an almost imperceptible sideward bend that makes the spine convex on its right side. Now "go with this movement" by putting the left hand on the lower rib cage from the left—the right hand is on the pelvis at the same time (fig. 9). It will ultimately become clear that the initial movement is equivalent to a shortening of the distance between the pelvic bone and the small ribs, with a corresponding side bend in the spine. These simultaneous movements of the hands should be produced easily.

Now hold the hands ready in place as before (the right one on the pelvis and the left on the lower rib cage, both on the pupil's left side) and watch the breathing movements. When

Fig. 9

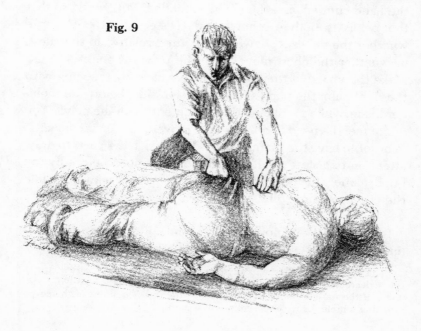

they are clearly visible, "go with" the *breathing-out* movement and help bring the pelvis and the rib cage closer to each other. This "help" should by no means be felt as an interference, but it may nevertheless prolong the exhalation and delay the next inhalation, the latter being deeper and slower than what might have been expected previously.

By this manipulon, the teacher substitutes his efforts for the efforts of the muscles connecting the ribs with the pelvis. These muscles, possibly by some excessive tension, are reducing the range of movement of the small ribs. With this substitution, these muscles are free to give up some of their tonus,* and the breathing mechanism, acting automatically (without the need of any conscious decision), immediately makes use of the latitude that has just been offered to it.

Now stand at the pupil's right side, facing the pelvis. Reach out with the left hand over the pupil's body and take hold of the left anterior superior spine from underneath, with the palm of the hand cupped, and the elbow extended. Pull gently so that the pelvis is both extended and twisted slightly. Observe whether the pelvis is allowed to be lifted relative to the chest, or whether the chest moves with the pelvis as one rigid unit. Make the image of the first alternative clear by touching with the right palm the pupil's ribs on the left side, below the shoulder blade, while producing the movements with the pelvis. You might feel the need to diminish the movement you are making, in order to have the thorax steady. Your touch then acts to draw attention to a state of affairs perhaps unnoticed before by the pupil, namely the possibility of moving one hip backward, while the chest remains still.

It might be useful now to review some of the practical guidelines that were outlined in the description of this series of

---

* This could be considered in a somewhat simplified way a *reversed* stretch reflex: decreased activity of muscle-length receptors during the "passive" shortening of the muscle reduces the activity of the motor neurons of the corresponding muscle, hence a lessening of the tonus.

manipulons. These guidelines and others will be helpful in the following chapters in establishing the tactics and the style of Functional Integration.

1. The movements are slow, nonintrusive, playing-checking-exploring, and the teacher, while looking for "obstacles," prefers easy adjustability. Repetitions are for clarification and familiarization.

2. Cardinal directions should be defined relative to the pupil's frame of reference, his adjustability being the center of interest.

3. With many movements there is a neutral position or section, not necessarily fixed forever, but somewhere within the range of each movement or between two "obstacles." A neutral position is a good starting point for moving in another cardinal direction.

4. As movement becomes easier it signifies a change in the pupil's representation and probably means that control is being taken over by a "higher" center.

5. Verbal remarks should be kept to a minimum and should relate to the representation of the distal parts moving in space. Emotionally loaded terms are to be avoided.

6. It is important to be aware of the limits of movement set by the structure of the joints.

7. The easy cooperation of proximal parts in the movements of distal parts should be regarded as a sign of efficiency.

8. A nondifferentiated movement, where two or more parts move as one unit, makes the *movement in space* familiar to the pupil, rendering an adequate representation possible. Also, the substitution of an outside effort for the effort of the muscles connecting these parts lessens their tonus. The succeeding differentiated movement, in which the parts move relative to each other, is then enhanced.

9. Force is applied in the direction of the intended movement, or adjusted to the direction of the resulting movement. If the movement (intended or resulting) is a rota-

tion, then the force should go with the movement in a direction tangential to the curve described. In producing movement, the direction and manner of applying force must be chosen with respect to adequacy, ease, and efficiency, without any preconception.

10. Many manipulons have some bearing on the breathing function in general or on a certain stage of the breathing cycle in particular. The teacher should not interfere inadvertently with the breathing movements, but should go, perhaps, *with* the breathing-out. Any deep breathing-in, once started, should be allowed completion. It might be a sign that some ongoing change is being acknowledged—perhaps not on a wholly conscious level—as being feasible, not endangering, and even releasing and beneficial.

11. It is useful to have at hand some criterion for judging the smallness of one's force. One example is given here: the force should compare with what is merely needed to shift the skin over its underlying bone or muscle.

12. A "parasitic" component of a movement can be cleared up by "going with it," exaggerating it slightly, then changing it to its opposite. Eventually, several possible alternatives are there to choose from, instead of a single "compulsive" one.

13. Identical movements produced on opposite sides of the body or in different positions are perceived in different contexts, and are therefore represented differently. That gives them an *integrative value,* by showing the pupil the manifold uses of *one* functional ability.

14. Touching a moving part (and "going with it"), or touching a muscle that participates in a movement—whether it is required for that movement or is superfluous—supplies the pupil with clear sensory information about that participation. This information eventually reaches higher (more conscious) levels in the brain, and helps to establish a more adequate representation of the action.

15. Changing the pattern of action involving a proximal joint may be facilitated by relating to the image of the involved distal limb moving in space; that is, relating to changes in the immediate environment.

16. A muscle fatigued by continuous activation and overtense will, if assisted by an "outside" force (be it some support, gravity, or the teacher's effort), ultimately lessen its tonus and thus movements heretofore hampered will be produced more easily.

4. A Classification of Manipulons

The reader now has a preliminary acquaintance with the style of Functional Integration and also an idea of the diversity of body structures as well as some knowledge of neuro-motor functions. With special awareness of this information and with a refined appreciation of the movements of his own body, he is now ready to consider a more detailed description of the nature of manipulons. As is the case with learning any new language, so will the learning of Functional Integration proceed from the simple repetition of basic phrases to engaging in meaningful body communication.

The classes of manipulons proposed and discussed further on are the following: (1) exploratory manipulons, (2) conforming manipulons, and (3) leading manipulons. Some of what I call the leading manipulons require an additional descriptive term, either because of a specific connotation they have or because of the context in which they appear. I will designate them *(a)* confining manipulons, *(b)* juxtaposing manipulons, *(c)* integrating manipulons, and *(d)* positioning manipulons.

1. Exploratory Manipulons

Exploratory manipulons serve to ask questions about the functioning of the neuro-muscular system and its relation to the structure of the bodily parts. Normally, they will precede any series of other manipulons. Information obtained by visual observation and initial conversation with the pupil is combined with the information obtained by exploratory manipulons to produce a coherent picture of the pupil's physical state. Any action that determines where, how, and to what degree a given force or pressure should be applied also constitutes an exploratory manipulon.

These exploratory touchings and handlings enrich the mental picture that the teacher already has of the pupil's *skeleton*. In this way the teacher gains a proper image of the skeletal structure concerning its placement, outline, and movability. The teacher must have this image in order to evaluate the quality of a movement, whether in observation only, or while producing a movement, and in order to know how to hold the body efficiently or to apply force—"force" being used as a physical concept, but not in the least suggesting magnitude or overpowering violence.

An obvious area of exploration is the elbow, where it is easy to locate the external and internal condyles of the humerus bone and the olecranon (elbow tip), which moves between them during flexion or extension of the elbow joint. The two condyles are convenient holding places of the arm in the elbow region, but also the origins (the sites of attachment) of the muscles involved in moving the hand and fingers—the external condyle serving as attachment for the extensors and the internal one for the flexors.

Another important area of exploration is, for example, the scapula. One can locate it easily by merely sliding a hand across its borders and feeling it through a garment. But a more efficient way of both locating the scapula and ascertaining its movability at the same time is the following: With the pupil lying on the stomach, the teacher places one hand over the area of the shoulderblade while using the other hand to lift the shoulder from underneath the shoulder joint. In this way not only will the outline of the scapula become clear, but one can systematically check the range of movements of the scapula; first laterally, by holding the outer and inner scapular borders with each hand and alternately sliding the scapula back and forth over the rib cage; secondly, by using both hands to push the superior and inferior scapular angles up and down; a third way is to grasp the spine of the scapula as one would a handle, sliding it over the rib cage at right angles to the spine.

Knowledge of the skeleton, its position, and the movements of its parts gives us an accurate description of the quality and range of movement from an external point of view. But such a description will not give us an unambiguous description of the pattern of muscular activity nor the pattern of action in the broader sense discussed in chapter 1. Appropriate use of exploratory manipulons gives us more direct information about the pupil's *muscular system,* which is the overt part of the effector system carrying out patterns of action. This exploration will reveal *(a) the latent muscular tonus,* a certain sustained tension in the musculature present even during inactivity and varying between flabbiness and spasticity—this constitutes the substrate for all muscular activity; *(b)* the various possible *modes of a muscle's participation* in movement patterns initiated by the teacher.

These various modes are in part determined by the character of the movement initiated, whether it is gentle or intrusive, carefully or awkwardly performed, slow or quick, expected or unexpected. It is the teacher who sets the style of the movements, guided by his own thinking and the ongoing sensory information. Different reactions can be sensed in the muscle's mode of participation in an induced movement: jerky contractions, a sudden slackening, a gradual increase or decrease of tension, or perhaps a total lack of activation. Moreover, depending on the context, the muscle may be expected to participate actively in producing the movement (in which case it is an agonist or synergist), or expected to be inactive, allowing the movement to occur (in which case it is an antagonist or opposing muscle). If the muscle is activated in spite of the fact that it is expected to rest, then it is a "parasitic synergist" whose superfluous effort must cease if the efficiency of the action is to increase.

One explores the way the muscle participates in a movement along these lines. The picture that emerges subsequently describes *a muscle's dynamic characteristic.* This term, however, merely denotes the perceivable display of what is occurring in the CNS in the course of its interaction with the immediate environment. The muscle's dynamic characteristic is not, then, an inherent attribute of the muscle.

Here is another exploratory procedure: With the pupil lying on the stomach, one touches one of the extensor muscles in the middle region of the back gently. One identifies its place and texture by sliding the fingers across the belly of the muscle—best done by gently shifting with flat fingers the pupil's skin to and fro—and then following it toward both its ends by longitudinal strokes on one side of the muscle and the other. One should identify the point at which the tendons of the muscle attach to the bone, palpating in a way that provides the best demonstration of the muscle's texture and its "dynamic characteristic." One may find that certain muscles, especially those of the limbs, are best explored by grasping the bulk of the muscle mass gently between thumb and fingers.

When one initiates a slight movement in order to discover the ease with which it is produced or the kind of reaction it elicits, one is performing an exploratory manipulon, and the reader will be able to identify such manipulations as described in chapter 3.

This exploration of ease of movement can also be done by adding to it the palpation of the involved muscle, in case its involvement is felt either as a help or as a hindrance to the attempted movement.

For example, while the pupil lies on the stomach, the teacher bends one of the lower legs with one hand by supporting it underneath the ankle, and with the other hand, palpates the hamstring muscles. Placing the hand on the muscle helps in exploring and discovering whether this is the muscle group that is helping in the flexion of the knee or interfering with the coming-down movement.

Sometimes it is useful, especially when this interference is quite pronounced, to put the pupil's hand on the involved muscle, and the pupil then gets the information directly through the sense of touch. For example, while the pupil is lying on his back with the head slightly rotated to one side—let's say to the right—it might happen that, with the slightest attempt of the teacher to lift the head off the table, the left sternocleido-mastoideus muscle (the left-side flexor of the neck) will simultaneously contract, and the reaction can be clearly seen. The pupil may become aware of the needless effort that is being made only through the sense of touch. One can ask him to use the fingers of the right hand to touch the muscle and then the information will come through this sense of touch, which is replacing for a while the kinesthetic sense. This might help in the discovery of the proprioceptive, kinesthetic sensation more clearly, which can then be used in controlling the muscle better.

A similar thing can be done by lifting the pupil's elbow while extending the upper arm and shoulder joint, while the fingers of the pupil's other hand touch the pectoral muscle and monitor its possibly excessive reaction.

Finding out the range of movement in a certain joint is, again, an exploratory manipulon. When done with utmost gentleness it enables one to find out in a sensory way whether the limits of the range of movement are set by the structure, such as the bones and ligaments that are part of the articulation, or by the muscular effort evoked by the pupil's nervous system.

While doing exploratory manipulons, one may encounter tense and string-like tendons, especially near the origin or the insertion of a muscle where the tendon is attached to the bone. Places like this could be quite sensitive to touch and should actually be left alone, although some clarification concerning the functions of the involved muscle (or its antagonist) might be indicated. Even gentle palpation of a tender spot might irritate it and should be avoided.

If something peculiar is *observed visually*, such as any peculiarity observed in walking, standing, or lying down, it should be taken into consideration. Details such as the distance of the arm and hands from the trunk, the direction in which the palms are facing, the equal or unequal amount of eversion of both feet as judged by the angles, should be noted. Any such particularity observed visually calls for an actual exploration by checking the appropriate movements. Only then will it become clear whether a peculiarity is there by chance and is, thus, transitory, or whether it constitutes a problem that should either be dealt with or left alone.

At certain more advanced stages of a session, one often checks the feasibility of initiating combined movements and one checks as well the reluctance or readiness of the pupil's system to allow such combined movements. This enables the teacher to evaluate the amount of control the pupil has over the motor system and also whether this control is enhancing adaptability.

For example, with the pupil on the back, the teacher places the left hand on the pupil's forehead and rolls the head slightly to the right and back to the middle. After this movement is done a few times, it can be combined with the lifting of the right scapula with the right hand, so that the rolling of the head to the right and the lifting of the right scapula up from the table are done simultaneously. A similar combination is also possible with the pupil lying on the side.

Another combined movement is the following: The pupil lies on the back, keeping the right elbow supported on the table and the forearm slightly lifted. The teacher produces simultaneously a slight extension of the elbow, a slight pronation of the forearm, and a slight extension of the wrist, a movement which could be summed up as bringing the base of the thumb slightly "down" (towards the foot).

Again, the pupil is on the back. The teacher holds his elbow and wrist up in the air, not fully extended. First, the entire arm is rotated so that the movement is in the shoulder joint. The rotation is then continued through the elbow so that the movements are in the shoulder joint and in the wrist.

This can be done in an analogous way with the leg and foot. The pupil lies on one side. The teacher slides the shoulder up and down and then adds to this the abduction of the elbow. One may try out two ways of combining: producing the abduction simultaneously with the sliding up of the shoulder or simultaneously with the down-slide.

2. Conforming Manipulons

With conforming manipulons the teacher joins in the pupil's movement completely, going along with what movement is allowed or initiated by the pupil. The conforming manipulons make the prevailing way of functioning clearer without challenging it. Instead, the prevailing function is accepted as one against which future changes will perhaps be compared. These manipulons set the ambience of "no danger" that is needed for a learning situation, and merely establish the pupil's representation of the habitual way of functioning. One has to inhibit the tendency to correct, and simply go with the pattern peculiar to the pupil.

The teacher will encounter one of two situations; one involving a "bias." If, for example, a bias is observed in posture or in the way of movement, one slightly increases this bias by facilitating it. For example, if, when the pupil lies on the back, the shoulders are involuntarily lifted off the table, one increases this bias by lifting them a little more or merely supporting them. Or, if both feet are everted differently, one helps the less everted to come to the middle. Or, if the head is flexed forward, whether in the supine or side position, this flexion is increased. Yet another example: if the pupil lies on the stomach and one observes a tendency to flex sidewards, then one helps by pulling the corresponding knee forward, flexing the corresponding arm, and positioning the hand in front of the face so that the pelvis and the shoulder girdle are elevated on the same side along with the lateral flexion.

The second situation occurs when a movement has been started and the teacher chooses to go in the direction that seems the easiest, selecting the frequency, speed, and range that seem to be most appropriate to the pupil's system. If a reaction is felt, one goes with that reaction. If a movement is repeated, one lets the "coming back" movement be done by the pupil's initiative or perhaps by gravity.

Examples of this are obvious. Here is one example connected with breathing movements: The pupil lies on his stomach, with the head turned to one side. One sits facing this side and observes the breathing movements. With the hands on the ribs, the teacher assists with the breathing-out movement, or helps the pelvis and the chest come nearer to each other accordingly.

When the breathing-in movement starts, one leaves the hands there, allowing it to happen, and goes again with the next breathing-out. One allows the rhythm to be set by the pupil's system.

3. Leading Manipulons

A leading manipulon usually grows out of a conforming manipulon, but incorporates some change in the pattern or in one component of the pattern. The change could be: *(a)* in the extent of movement, by making it slightly bigger or smaller; *(b)* in the direction of the movement, by leading the movement in a direction slightly different from the habitual one; *(c)* in the speed of movement, by making it faster or slower; *(d)* in the rhythm, by changing a regular movement to an irregular one or vice versa, or changing the rhythm of a regular repetitive movement to a faster or a slower one; *(e)* adding or subtracting, covertly or overtly, a movement element, thus making it different from the habitual; *(f)* adding some sensory input that might not have been perhaps so clear before, such as touching a moving part or touching a muscle that is expected to participate differently than it does, that is, more gradually or perhaps not at all; *(g)* repeating a pattern that was already done, but in a new constellation, a new position, or a new set of circumstances, so that the habitual pattern or response is less likely to occur.

Examples of these have already appeared in chapter 3, and are easily recognizable as such. In terms of repeating a pattern *(g)*, initiating any combined movement could be an example. For instance, the pupil lies on the back and a movement made previously with the pupil's arm is now produced while supporting the scapula in an appropriate way so that it now participates in the movement of the arm and the rolling of the head. Another example is to put a hard roller underneath the knees and another one behind the ankles (the pupil is lying on the back), so that the legs can easily roll to the sides, or at least be felt as ready to roll easily. The teacher pushes or pulls slightly through the head in the direction of the pelvis, or away from it.

Another example: The pupil is in the same position as before with rollers underneath his legs, and the soles of the feet are pushed alternately or simultaneously in the direction of the head. Eventually the head may start rocking as it is pulled and pushed by the spinal movements. It is important in the two last examples that the force is gently propagated through the skeleton.

(a) Confining Manipulons

A confining manipulon is a special kind of leading manipulon where the change limits a movement range, either of movements done as a reaction to some pattern or of breathing movements or of movements that are expected to occur. A confining manipulon calls for a changed way of adaptation or of programming, because of a change in the immediate environment.

Limiting a movement range is not always seen as a negative occurrence for the pupil. Sometimes a manipulon provides a substitute for the habitual effort of the pupil's own system, so that this system finds a way making good use of it. This is done either by some structural support or by pressure from the teacher's hands. Sometimes a manipulon puts a rigid obstacle against the moving part, and sometimes it is only a touch that suggests a limiting of the available space.

A confining manipulon should always leave an "escape" open, and should not be felt as intruding. In other words, it should limit from one side only, and leave open possibilities of movement in the other direction.

Many examples will be encountered in subsequent chapters, but a few should be described here.

A roller put underneath the knees, while the pupil is on the back, will free the pupil from worrying about hyperextending the knees, which might sometimes be stressed or even painful.

Soft rollers, two inches in diameter, which are put longitudinally underneath the shoulder joint will relieve some of the effort of the pectoral muscles. A similar thing can be done with the flexors of the neck by putting a support underneath the neck or the back of the head in order to limit any possible hyperextension of the neck.

A support, although limiting movement, might simultaneously be felt to be providing safety and comfort. A typical confining manipulon will be a movement done by the teacher in one direction only. There it stops; it does not initiate the coming-back movement. The position is held until the pupil's CNS takes it as a change in the environment that demands a corresponding adaptation and change in the pattern of movement.

This holding-in-support goes on sometimes for a few seconds only, sometimes more, until the changed reaction of the pupil's system is felt. This can be a change in tonus in a certain muscle group, or a breathing-in movement. In any case, if such an adaptive change occurs, it is to be considered as "accepted" by the pupil.

A second example: While the pupil lies on the stomach, the teacher presses very gently on the crown of the head in the direction of the upper cervical vertebrae (along the tangent of the cervical curve, at the uppermost vertebra), holds this for a few seconds, then releases. Now one presses the sole of the foot through the extended leg so that the pelvis does a very small rotation and holds this a few seconds (the pupil can be prone or supine). The exact direction of the pressure, the orientation of the leg, and the preliminary rotation of the leg required for this manipulon must be explored beforehand.

Similarly, with the pupil lying on the back, one can press on the rim of the pelvic bone so that the pelvis flexes very slightly. This position is held for a few seconds.

Next one presses very gently on the ribs on one side of the trunk, as if to interfere with the breathing-in movement, and holds this position for five to ten seconds.

(b) Juxtaposing Manipulons

A juxtaposing manipulon presents two differing states of affairs, so that the pupil can evaluate the difference. The difference may already have been present or may have been produced after clarifying the movement on one side. It often leads to emphasizing an aspect of a movement pattern, such as the amount of effort needed to perform the same movements on both sides, whether this be done by the pupil or by the teacher. It may also provide a comparison of the range of two movements.

Juxtaposing manipulons usually contrast the left side with the right side of the body. The insight gained by this shows the pupil what is really happening and can be helpful in transferring the program from the more satisfactory side to the deficient one. In one-sided paresis (partial paralysis) the pupil needs to understand how much relative effort is really needed, and the juxtaposition of the two sides can show effectively what is expected from the affected side.

Not only can left and right sides be contrasted, but also two successively performed patterns of movement make a comparison possible for the pupil, provided attention is drawn to it. An example of the latter could be as follows: Show the pupil how to rotate the head to the side in two ways, one with the chin 'tucked in, and the other with the chin away from the throat. In short, two similar patterns are presented, emphasizing one aspect in two different ways. The pupil compares these different ways in the representation, thus improving the ability to control these patterns equally.

Sometimes the mere checking of one aspect of a pattern on both sides, after some clarification has been done on one of the sides, may be enough for the pupil to comprehend the juxtaposition without the teacher having to draw attention to it verbally.

(c) Integrating Manipulons

What makes a leading manipulon into an integrating one is the fact that it has been preceded by other manipulons in which a specific element has been clarified and is now approached in a different manipulatory context.

It is possible that a new pattern will only be perceived by the pupil as a transient experience, without having any lasting bearing on his everyday patterns. But this unwanted event need not happen: the more any new pattern or one of its elements is felt to be *connected with as many other functions as possible,* the more it will have a chance to be integrated and assimilated into the pupil's normal way of acting.

The change introduced in the pupil's representation by this kind of leading manipulon will serve to supplement and complete the pupil's image of the ongoing activity, either by *drawing his attention to certain aspects* or details that might be obscure, thus turning them into clear parts of the pattern, or by changing the context (the immediate environment, the orientation, the goal of the activity). In other words, the new representation will *extend the series of patterns* connected with the *same* element that was clarified before.

Now follow a few examples of integrating manipulons. Suppose the pupil lies on one side with the head supported and the knees drawn up slightly, and one applies pressure through the neck in the direction of the pelvis, and makes the pelvis move slightly (as described in chapter 3). One can now consider the movability of the pelvis as a "new element" that calls for further integration. Continuing with one hand pushing through the neck, one puts the other hand on the pelvis. This integrating manipulon draws the attention of the pupil to the new element. Then one pushes the pelvis upwards, which again highlights the same element in a different context.

For a further series of integrating manipulons connected with the above-mentioned "new element," one has the pupil sitting. One then pushes either buttock up (perhaps from underneath the greater trochanter), so that the pelvis tilts slightly to the side and the shoulder on the same side moves down. The same movability of the pelvis can be now checked with movements for looking up or looking down (the pupil is still sitting), or looking backwards over one of the shoulders.

(d) Positioning Manipulons

A positioning manipulon is one that arranges the pupil's body in a given position or helps change this position when needed. These positions are determined by two factors: the pupil's *comfort* and the *plan* of the forthcoming manipulations.

If there is any disability or pain limiting the pupil's movement, this should be taken into consideration in choosing a suitable posture. *Paddings* and *supports* should not be spared. In most instances, a more or less flexed position is easier than an extended one, a straight position easier than a twisted one.

The position should allow some movement of those parts that the teacher is interested in checking first. Obviously, there is more than one solution to this, so that the choice should be made taking into consideration both factors (the pupil's comfort and the teacher's didactical intentions), while allowing also for subsequent variations.

Many times, the pupil could simply be asked to assume a given position, but the teacher has to decide if this might not be too difficult or extreme for any particular pupil. If this is the case, then it is appropriate to offer help, especially in changing from one position to another.

For example, with the pupil on the stomach, and the head turned to one side, one has to make sure that the twist in the cervical spine is not uncomfortable. The best way of easing the position (in case the prone position is required) is to draw up the corresponding leg: one takes the ankle with one hand in order to flex the knee slightly, then one takes the knee with the other hand and rotates the thigh in a slight outward rotation, while sliding the knee up. One can leave the knee midway and transfer the hand to help the pelvis from underneath, so that it adjusts easily to this slightly twisted state, an action which partly straightens the neck. The corresponding arm is flexed forward to support a similar lifting of this side of the shoulder girdle, and the other arm is placed alongside the body.

Eventually the need will arise to change the position of the head over to the other side. The teacher will proceed with the appropriate positioning manipulon in a logical way by gently straightening out the bent leg and bringing the straight arm forward. One has to check that both shoulders are not pressed down too much and that both forearms are not too far from the trunk, so that the pupil will be ready to utilize them for support. The teacher now puts both hands around the base of the pupil's head, so that one hand is around the back of the skull and the other around the base of the jaw. In this way the thumbs are above and the fingers underneath the head. The head can now be lifted, only as much as is needed to tuck in the chin slightly, and its turn completed. Care must be taken not to extend the head and not to increase the twist in the neck. One might feel the need to stop in the middle of the procedure and, with the head supported with both hands, to check whether there is any bias left or right before going on with the turn.

The reader may design a positioning manipulon for changing over from the supine position to the prone, and vice versa.

Sometimes through a positioning manipulon the pupil learns something new about personal spatial relationships within the environment, about possible comfortable postures, and about efficiency in moving.

Some of the manipulons presented in this chapter may be self-explanatory as to their purpose or intended result. Others may, for the moment, seem only to be slightly different styles of manipulons. The reasons for using the latter manipulons as well as their expected outcomes will be clarified in the next chapter.

5. The Various Modes of the Pupil's Response: The Limbic and Cortical Levels of Control

We shall now survey the manipulons once again, this time concentrating on the reaction of the pupil. In practice, the teacher of Functional Integration notices two major levels of control and reaction on the part of the pupil. These two levels are generally related to what in neuro-physiology are called the limbic and cortical systems. I shall not go into the precise definition and localization in the brain of these systems; for our purposes it suffices to differentiate these two levels from the functional viewpoint.

It is an important fact that all levels of control share the same effector system, namely, the cerebrospinal tract, the motor nerves, the muscles, and the skeleton. This explains the fact that even though shifting control from one level to the other is possible, there is never a simultaneous sharing of control of the same motor units. I cannot yawn and chew at the same time, anymore than I can breathe in while hiccuping. Another example: If someone stretches out the arm to reach for something and suddenly hears a loud, startling noise, he will withdraw the arm in a defensive movement, interrupting the intentional movement that had been started. Obviously, a lower level of control has intervened, stimulated by the unexpectedness of the startling sensation.

Thus the two levels of control, limbic and cortical, are mutually exclusive. A similar instance occurs when a person with spasticity, tremor, or some other neuro-motor disturbance learns to control it by slowly and deliberately performing a goal-directed movement with the affected body parts. In such an action, the upper level has taken over the effector system and thus inhibits a pattern otherwise controlled by the lower level. As soon as a pupil is made to realize that there are two (or even more) such alternatives, a choice may be made and acting by compulsion may cease.

The lower level manifests its control and initiates activity in the following areas:

1. in hereditary reflexes
2. in conditions of danger when quick defensive reactions are evoked
3. in early-achieved motor patterns such as antigravity mechanisms
4. in emotionally loaded actions
5. in states of regression such as occur after trauma or disease
6. where there are neurological deficiencies, whether peripheral or central
7. where there is pain

Feldenkrais has come to refer to the lower level of control as "the idiot within us."

The upper level of control manifests itself in quite different functions:

1. in selecting single strands of information from a muddle of noise
2. in exploring, such as the way in which an infant learns about its immediate environment
3. in asking questions
4. in comparing things, experiences, ideas, possibilities of action
5. in playing games, acting, teasing

6. in performing refined, intentional actions
7. in programming intentional, goal-directed activities
8. in a "meta-attitude" toward any activity, namely, the act of "looking at" an ongoing activity

It must be remembered that any upper-level activity may be taken over by a lower level if conditions suddenly require an immediate response or, in a different fashion, if a person is lulled gradually into habitual, stereotypical behavior. In some instances "the idiot within us" proves itself to be quicker or more dominant.

It is important to note that the teacher of Functional Integration is able to sense the level of control in the pupil by the way in which the pupil responds to the exploratory manipulons. This possibility opens the way for helping the pupil raise the level of control from the limbic to the cortical spheres.

Let us now return to the subject of teacher-pupil interaction. During any manipulon, especially those that are exploratory, one usually feels that one is communicating with the pupil's upper level of control—one is, in a sense, "talking" to a responsible person. In this instance, what previously was unclear to the pupil has become more obvious. In most cases this occurs in patterns involving the upper part of the body, head, arms, and hands. At this point, depending on the teacher's skill and imagination, the pupil's experience can be enriched with a few new patterns of movement, either those needed for some special task or simply those that will expand the pupil's repertoire of skills.

A more interesting possibility is for the teacher to address "the idiot within" the pupil directly. By constantly noting the continuous feedback of sensory response during the manipulons, the teacher restricts the "conversation" to stereotyped reactions characteristic of lower-level control. In most cases, as will be explained in this chapter, these are patterns of action affecting the trunk, back, pelvis, and legs. Sometimes these patterns may be initiated by emotional, or internal, visceral stimuli. Such reactions may well be determined by pathological states or processes as well as by inherited, instinctive patterns, or those learned early in life. In either case they will be acted out by habit in a more or less automatic way and are clearly not goal-directed, intentional actions.

To help the pupil overcome this situation and attain a higher level of control, the teacher has to address the lower level in its own language; to create *new* situations in which the pupil's lower-level system responds in its typical way. Such an occurrence being new to the pupil's experience, the response may now differ from the stereotypical behavior. This new awareness, which betokens a higher level of control, may then be integrated into the pupil's system.

By surveying some of the characteristic ways in which lower-level control operates, it will become clearer how we can effectively address these lower levels.

1. Working Through Antagonists

The muscles producing opposite movements, such as flexion and extension, are called agonists and antagonists (remember, by the way, that either one can be considered the antagonist of the other). In joints displaying such muscular dyads there is a reciprocal functional organization, which insures that the activation of one of the two muscles goes together with the inhibition of its antagonist. This Sherringtonian principle of reciprocal inhibition is controlled via *(a)* low-level involuntary neural connections in the ventral horn of the spinal cord and *(b)* central connections carrying descending impulses from the cortex to the lower spinal neurons—this latter usually being a higher, voluntary level.

One can demonstrate to oneself this phenomenon of reciprocal inhibition by simply bending the right forearm and holding something heavy in the palm of the right hand. Using the fingers of the left hand to feel the upper muscles of the right arm, one will feel that the biceps is taut and that the triceps—

the antagonist on the backside of the upper arm—will be soft. Of course one *can* also make the triceps taut but only by the additional voluntary effort of, for example, imagining that one is making one's entire arm stiff. Conversely, if one presses the palm of the right hand downward on a table, elbow bent, the triceps will be taut and the biceps will be soft. But one can discover another interesting neuro-muscular fact if one presses down on the table's surface this time with the back of the hand. In this situation both the biceps and the triceps will be taut because the biceps is now being used to supinate the forearm, that is, to turn the forearm on its axis so that the palm faces upwards.

In other important joints we find more complex movements such as this, movements involving more than a simple dyad of back-and-forth-motion. The knee joints are similar to the elbow in this respect. Similar complex movements are found in the wrists, ankles, hip joints, and shoulder joints, all of which are universal joints that allow movement in all planes, including rotation around the limb's axis. Also the movements of the scapulae, the jaw, and particularly the spinal column involve more than simple flexion and extension. The lumbar and cervical vertebrae, for example, can allow both lateral bending and twisting simultaneously while engaged in either flexion or extension.

If movement patterns around a joint are habitual and under lower-level control, then any variation in the simple agonist-antagonist movement must involve control at the higher level. Variations such as change from an habitual direction, speed, or range requires the operation of the higher level. In such instances the pupil either voluntarily performs a different movement or is able to allow it to be performed by someone else. Such voluntary actions are one of the preliminary steps in programming new patterns of movement in the pupil.

The simple action of exploring the relationship between two antagonists can, in itself, improve the pupil's control, because it may clarify in the pupil's own awareness the function of reciprocal inhibition. If the pupil has difficulty releasing a tense muscle involuntarily, the teacher can involve this muscle in a different pair of opposing movements. In an altered movement pattern the balky muscle may very well have behaved normally and, working from this new point of freedom, the teacher can gradually restore the previously hampered function of the original antagonists.

An example of the above would be to have the pupil lying on his stomach while the teacher holds the ankle and attempts to flex and straighten the knee. It may be discovered that the pupil cannot release the hamstring muscles so that the foot can come down. If this is the case, the following manipulon could be tried: holding the ankle with both hands, while the knee is bent and the foot slightly raised, turn the heel toward the outside and then back toward the middle line until an easy rotation of the leg occurs in both the knee and hip joint. This rotation creates an alternating movement in the hamstrings, differentiating them more clearly. Then, by slightly lowering the leg during the outward turn of the heel, the pupil will experience the pattern of letting the foot come down.

This same procedure can be used in cases of more serious disturbance. The change may be slow, however, in which case other approaches to be described later should be employed.

Two typical situations of a more serious nature occur when both agonist and antagonist are simultaneously tense (spasticity) or when one is tense and the other is not used at all. These and similar situations usually stem from peripheral or central damage (of congenital, traumatic, or degenerative origin) to the nervous system. Only after considerable experience can the teacher hope to be of help with such disturbances (see chapter 10).

2. Antigravitational Patterns and the Efficient Use of the Skeleton

Like all other bodies on earth, we are continuously subjected to the downward pull of gravity. The persistence of this force throughout the phylogenetic history of our species and throughout our personal lives makes certain that our CNS has antigravitational patterns thoroughly ingrained in its functions. This, of course, means that they are under low-level control and are carried out automatically without our volition. Any movement, no matter how small, may provoke an adaptive response to gravity and, indeed, the motor system is almost continually involved in such responses. To say *anti*gravitational is a bit misleading, because we don't always fight against gravity but frequently turn it to our advantage by using our upright posture and thus the body's high potential energy for an easy, pendulum-like initiation of movement, or using gravity-produced friction to stop movement. As we know, there are only a few situations when our CNS is freed from its concern with gravity: one of these is in space flight, when gravity is balanced out by inertial forces, or when the body is immersed in a fluid whose specific gravity equals the body's mean specific gravity. The floating of a fetus within the amniotic fluid is an example of the latter.

There is one situation that simulates this neutralization of gravity: it is the act of lying down on a horizontal surface, a position which provides the sensation of being securely supported. This not only frees the person from the need for activating the antigravity muscles, most of which are extensors, but it also reduces the adaptive relevance of incoming sensory information in relation to gravity. This is to say that the horizontal position diminishes the alertness of the CNS to information which otherwise would stimulate a continuous adaptive response to gravity.

There are several sensory modalities involved in postural adaptation to the field of gravity: the vestibular apparatus, located in the inner ear, which informs us of head position in relation to verticality and acceleration; the proprioceptive sense organs in the muscles, tendons, and joints, which inform us of muscular position and effort; the exteroceptive sense organs of the skin, which are sensitive to immediate pressures outside the body; the interoceptive senses in the inner organs, which affect posture and muscular behavior; and the teleceptors, which sense at a distance. The latter include the visual, auditory, and olfactory receptors. Usually there are no contradictory responses to these variegated incoming stimuli, because the CNS integrates this afferent information and only one efferent system of impulses reaches the effectors.

The horizontal position frees all of these sensory modalities from their usual antigravitational responses. Instead, there is a condition of ease, reduced muscular tonus, and usually a greater degree of higher-level control. This condition makes possible the evocation of nonstereotyped patterns of action that can subsequently be used in a standing position.

Antigravitational patterns should be looked at from two viewpoints: *(a)* the patterns of muscular effort and coordination, such as activation of extensor muscles versus flexors, and *(b)* the efficiency with which the skeletal structure is used. The importance of the latter becomes apparent even from the most elementary consideration of the dynamic functions of the human skeleton, which is a complex system of levers that have different forces acting upon them: the gravitational forces of the body on its parts, forces from objects coming in contact with the body (such as weight, and frictional and elastic forces), and muscular forces. The supportive functions of the skeleton usually occur without the person being aware of the essential role performed by the skeleton's rigidity. Instead of looking at these functions only from a kinesiological viewpoint, we should pay attention to the amount of muscular effort or fatigue involved in efficient or inefficient use of the skeleton.

Another aspect of the skeleton's function concerns the rigidity of the bony structure in transmitting forces through the bones along their axes. If only one bone is involved in transmission of force, we do not need to be concerned, but if two or more bones are conjoined in transmitting force then the alignment of the joints becomes of crucial importance. Obviously, when the joints connecting the bones are nearer to a straight line in the act of transmitting force, the muscular effort needed to stabilize these joints is smaller. When the joints are aligned straight, all effort is, in principle, at zero, the force being taken over by the bony structure itself rather than the muscles. A simple example will suffice to illustrate this: Compare the degree of muscular effort needed to push or pull a heavy object with a hand, when the elbow is slightly bent, with the degree of effort for the same action with a fully straightened elbow. In the latter case the effort is performed by the larger muscles of the trunk while the arm muscles relax, thus providing a feeling of ease and efficiency in performing the action.

Efficient use of the skeleton involves important antigravitational functions. For example, to go from a sitting to an upright position recruits various antigravitational muscles, mainly the extensors. But once the vertical stance is attained, the effort of the extensors can be given up almost completely. This condition is, in fact, a basic criterion for efficient verticality, the bones and joints being aligned in a manner that allows the weight of the body to be borne by the skeleton. In this state the muscles and the complex system controlling them are disengaged from the responsibility of maintaining the upright posture and become freed for other actions. This freedom and the concomitant readiness for action is a precondition for actualizing the several advantages of the erect human posture.

These advantages should be mentioned at least briefly.

Skeletal support allows an easy turning of the head around a vertical axis so that the person can scan the surroundings and turn toward an interesting or dangerous outside stimulus that has reached the teleceptors (eyes, ears, and nostrils).

The turning (rotating) of the body around its vertical axis, in order to align it with the turned head or for any other purpose, is made easy, quick, and effort-saving by the fact that in this position the "moment of inertia" of the body with respect to that axis is small, compared with other possible postures. More simply stated, the nearer to the axis of rotation the mass of a rotating body is distributed, the easier it is to initiate or to stop the body's rotation.

The center of gravity of the human body being in its highest position, the potential energy is also highest. Statically considered, this is an "unstable equilibrium," the center of gravity being high and the supporting surface small. But notwithstanding this, when it is considered *dynamically*, the erect posture is a most efficient starting point for movement. A small deviation from the vertical doesn't call for any special effort. It initiates a "losing" of balance, which is easily recovered by an appropriate movement of the pelvis and legs. Hence, walking about on a horizontal surface becomes an easy, gliding movement. There is, in other words, readiness for action without the need for preliminary preparation.

Finally, the sense of support provided by the skeleton elicits a lowering of the muscular tonus all over the system, therefore enhancing flexibility, lightness, and vitality. There is also a continuous neurological vigilance (not necessarily conscious) in having underlying support for the body's weight. The moment the firmness of support is felt, the weight of the body rests upon it with the muscles relaxing accordingly. Most of these responses become habitual early in life and are therefore effected through lower-level control.

A comparison of this ideal vertical situation with the actual performance of different individuals, or of the same person at different times and in different situations, shows that the most efficient use of the skeleton does not always occur. For example, when the flexors of the trunk are activated, as part of an intentional pattern of flexing, then the corresponding extensors (the antagonists) will usually slacken. But the flexors (of the hips, the pelvis, or the neck) can be activated as part of other patterns too, as in defensive postures, when there is anxiety or pain, or simply out of habit. This will require the simultaneous activation of the extensors to prevent bending. A vicious circle of reciprocal stimulation and reinforcement of the antagonist muscle pairs is thus the result, and it causes a lack of flexibility, an inefficient use of the skeleton, antigravitational actions produced with superfluous effort, and tiredness. Bringing higher-level control into play can show the pupil a way out of this situation.

Manipulons that are relevant to situations such as this have already been described, and others will be mentioned in later chapters. For working through the skeleton and providing the sensation of forces being transmitted throughout, see, for example, the last manipulons described in the section "Leading Manipulons" in chapter 4.

3. Movements of the Extremities Versus Trunk Movements

The limbs (the distal body parts) have a *greater movement range* than the larger (proximal) parts of the body, and this makes the representation of the actions of the distal parts clearer for the pupil and easier to monitor. The possible movements of the distal parts are also more complex than those of the proximal parts, because more articulations are involved. For example, the shoulder moves more in extent and in variety than the chest, the elbow more than the shoulder, and the wrist more than the elbow. The same applies to the legs and feet.

It is therefore safe to assume, for that reason, that the extremities (the limbs) are controlled more by the upper level of the brain, and the trunk more by the lower level. This situation creates the possibility of using familiar patterns of movement in which the trunk is involved in an intentional movement of a limb, in order to clarify the participation of the proximal part in this movement and, hence, in other movements as well.

It often happens that the representation of a proximal-movement pattern fades away with time and, with it, the movement itself. A leading manipulon emphasizing or enhancing this proximal part of the pattern, such as the movement of the scapula while acting with the hand and arm, or the movement of the pelvis while moving the leg (bending, rotating, and the like) will supply the pupil with the image of increasing the range of movement and of doing it with greater ease, having experienced the bigger muscles being used synergetically rather than adversely.

Clarifications of this kind can restore or increase the flexibility of the trunk, and specifically the connection between the pelvis and the thorax, where the lower level of control usually prevails. A few manipulons that may serve this purpose have already been described, and more may be devised by an inventive teacher. Other manipulons will be presented in subsequent chapters.

4. Relative Conjugate Movements

The image representing a pattern of movement contains a frame of reference, in relation to which movements are carried out and perceived. This frame of reference can be either the surrounding space and be represented by nearby objects, or more intimately, by parts of the body itself. Compare, for example, turning your head to the right in order to look at an object situated there, with a similar turning of the head for the purpose of looking at a speck on the backside of your right shoulder. These movements, objectively the same, are defined by two different frames of reference. Sometimes both aspects are there, intermingled and alternating, as in walking or climbing stairs. In examples such as these, we are usually quite aware both of the movement of our body relative to the immediate surrounding and the movement of parts of the body relative to each other.

It will be useful to distinguish two special cases. Consider two parts of the body in relation to each other, with one part moving relative to the immediate surrounding, while the other is stationary. This situation involves *two* different patterns of movement that have a methodically significant relationship. We will call them "relative conjugate movements." One of the two has a distal and lighter part moving, while the neighboring proximal and heavier part is motionless. This is usually a clear, even if habitual pattern, easily accessible to conscious (upper-level) control. The other pattern has a proximal (heavy) part moving relative to a stationary distal part, and this pattern may be less clear to envisage and thus difficult to perform by the pupil.

A manipulon that has a distal part fixed in space and the respective proximal part moving is, therefore, likely to clarify difficult patterns of action and to increase the differentiation of movements. But the real importance of relative conjugate movements is that they offer another way of teaching how to work around certain functional difficulties.

Let us stop for a moment to discuss a particular characteristic of *voluntary* patterns of movement.

When a voluntary action is performed, the sensory systems in the CNS that will receive the sensory impulses pertaining to that action are already preset for the consequences of these actions. In other words, the centers processing sensory information receive impulses from the cerebral motor system (the intentional cortex), so that the incoming sensory information related to the performed action is at least partly expected. Such a mechanism of anticipatory motor-to-sensory flow of impulses is termed by some neuro-physiologists "corollary discharge," and by others "efference-copy."

This anticipatory mechanism, which is not active during an involuntary (reflex) action or during an environment-produced action, serves several purposes. One is to guarantee the *invariance* of the spatial order of perception while performing movements. Here is a classic example: Moving the eyes (with or without moving the head) changes the place on the retina of the images of objects in the visual field, but nevertheless these are *perceived* as being steady. A vertical line, for example, will be *perceived as vertical,* even while tilting the head from side to side. On the other hand, if you simply push your eyeball sideways with a finger—this is an utterly *unhabitual* way of turning the eye—you will see the visual field jump. In this case, the anticipatory information about the movement of the eye is lacking, while in the former case such information, stemming from the motor center as *part of the voluntary motor pattern,* brings about a compensation which takes place while processing the visual information in the brain. This processing has the effect of preserving the spatial order of perception. The question as to how this invariance is produced and how the processing of information in the visual centers yields visual perception still awaits detailed answers. Similar examples may be found for other sensory modalities.

Another function of this anticipatory mechanism is to *inhibit* or to change the usual reaction to a sensory stimulus, in the case of the stimulus being the consequence of a self-produced, voluntary action. If I touch myself on the back, with my hand or with a stick, it won't occur to me to turn around to see who is touching me.

These anticipatory processes, which occur with self-produced actions and their relationship to the perception of the environment (the person's own body included), can be and are learned. They are also adaptable to changed or distorted conditions. Suppose I descend a ladder that has its rungs equally spaced. If somewhere down the ladder one of the rungs happens to be spaced differently from the others I might get a jolt, or if the space is greater, I might feel I had lost my footing, for a split second at least. This shows that I have *learned* to anticipate the sensations that accompany my movements.

It is plausible to assume that processes of this kind are learned from early childhood and have an important role in developing sensory-motor coordination, voluntary control of action, and gradual differentiation between the self and the non-self (the environment).

Anticipatory motor-to-sensory discharges could have, in certain circumstances, a functionally restricting effect. Consider the case of a person who experiences discomfort or pain while making a certain movement. Whatever the origin of such discomfort, structural or functional, a few repetitions of the movement will render the anticipation of that pain an integral part of the pattern. In other words, the mere consideration of doing the movement is colored, in that person's mind, with such an anticipation. Obviously, this will limit the readiness to use that pattern and will even create "anti-patterns," thus activating antagonists concomitantly as soon as there is any attempt to produce the movement. Strangely enough, all of these avoidances and defenses usually exceed by far what is really necessary. Moreover, these anti-patterns can persist as habits, even after the defensive need for them is diminished or entirely gone. They have become, in other words, "low-level" controlled.

The relative conjugate movement, gently proposed by the teacher, is designed to be free of such linkage. Its pattern has a different spatial orientation; it is related to a different representation and to a different context, and the level of clarity is different. Anti-patterns might be aroused, if at all, by the *newness* of the proposed pattern, but not by anticipated sensations of pain or discomfort. Sensations of the latter kind are not expected. The teacher will by no means produce pain by this kind of manipulon, if he maintains the right style of manipulation. In this way, the pupil learns through his senses the ease, the extent (however small), and the feasibility of movements in a certain joint with certain muscles. The surprise comes when the teacher leads the pupil back gradually to the original, inhibited movement. "Gradually" means, of course, adding some movement to the distal part and decreasing the movement of the proximal part that was involved in the relative conjugate movement, thus transforming the pattern into the very one which was previously avoided.

On the other hand, if a particular movement triggers a sense of inability or weakness (but not necessarily pain), then the anticipated feeling of impotence might evoke substitute efforts from the stronger and abler parts of the motor system, efforts that will make up for the deficient muscular contractions. This not only deviates from the initially intended movement, but also prevents possible use of the weaker, impaired parts of the body—the way to regeneration or relearning is blocked. Sometimes it is possible to coach such a person to give up the misdirected efforts and to look for the "something" lacking by employing *very slight* efforts. But sometimes, also, a relative conjugate movement can help circumvent the expectation of failure, thus opening the way for exploring and developing new possibilities.

A few examples will be helpful in clarifying the technique of relative conjugate movements: Take an example involving movements of the hip joint. Let the pupil lie on the stomach, the head turned to the left. Sit near the left side, facing the pupil's left thigh. Bend the left knee at a right angle by holding the left leg near the ankle and lifting it up. Then bring the ankle slightly towards you to the left. This will produce an inward rotation of the thigh. Now bring it back to the vertical position. Repeat this a few times to acquaint yourself, as well as the pupil, with the quality of the movement. In many cases you will find that the range of movement is less than the possible range; something stops the movement before it comes to its structural limit. Now do the relative conjugate movement: Continuing to hold the bent leg stationary in space (that is, vertical) with your right hand, make the pelvis rotate slightly by slipping your left hand (or fist) underneath it somewhere between the pelvic crest and the left greater trochanter so that the left side of the pelvis is somewhat lifted up. Then let it return to the original position. If this movement is resisted, then you can clarify the pupil's understanding through the movement of the more distal body part, by simultaneously rotating the thigh outward (holding the leg near the ankle), so that both your hands push slightly away from you. After a few repetitions of this "nondifferentiated movement" (the thigh and the pelvis moving as one piece), you can gradually turn it into a "differentiated movement" by continuing the movement of the pelvis and diminishing the movement of the leg, until the latter can be kept vertically steady.

Thus, the relative conjugate movement becomes accepted as a feasible pattern and, along with it, there is a changed context of expectation in the use of the hip joint. To help in integrating that change, you should gradually turn that movement into the inhibited movement tried at first. You may then discover, together with the pupil, an increased range of movement with a different quality and a different level of control.

Take an example related to the shoulder joint. The pupil lies on the left side, knees drawn up comfortably, the head on an appropriate soft support. Lift the pupil's right elbow away from the side (lateral abduction of the humerus). If there is resistance, try the relative conjugate movement, in order to make clear whether the difficulty is mainly functional and can be bypassed in this manner. Grasp the bent right elbow in your left hand and lift it up in abduction, but only to a small degree easily acceptable to the pupil. Grasp the shoulder joint with the right hand (between thumb and fingers), so that the palm applies its surface to the pupil's shoulder. With the upper arm securely between the hands, move it alternately up and down (toward the head and toward the pelvis). Even the smallest movement will do. At the beginning, don't increase the distance between the elbow and trunk. By gently repeating the movement, you may find that with every push of the shoulder the elbow moves slightly away from the trunk. Maintain this new distance while coming back: the distance will gradually increase until the elbow extends vertically above the shoulder; then you can move the shoulder while keeping the elbow stationary in space.

Here is another example with the pupil lying on his side. Moving the upper chest forward (or backward) while keeping the pelvis stationary (rotation of the spine), or, conversely, moving the pelvis in this way while the chest is kept motionless, constitute two relative conjugate movements. It is a good practice to explore both options to determine which one is less connected with anticipations that call for defenses, and, after having established one secure pattern, to utilize the other one.

Or, let the pupil lie on the back with knees drawn up, so that the feet are planted on the bench as in standing. Sit facing the toes of the right leg. Grasp with your left hand the right leg near the ankle, so that you can keep the leg steady, or at least emphasize by this the fact that it is going to remain fixed during the movement. With the fingers of your right hand find the navicular bone (the prominent bone on the medial side of the instep). Support it from underneath, where the arch of the foot is highest, and push it up diagonally in the direction of your own left wrist, for example. Since the sole of the foot is being held in place, the result is a displacement of the ankle to the outside with some lateral bending, which constitutes the relative conjugate movement of what is called "inversion of the foot." The degree of the movement to be made and its appropriate direction are easily found, provided this is done in the exploratory style already discussed.

A much more delicate example is related to movements of the head and neck. One should attempt this only if sure of the delicacy of one's touch. With the pupil lying supine, put an appropriate flat support beneath the head if needed, so that there will be no extra strain in the neck muscles. Sit facing the pupil's head from above. Put your left palm horizontally on the forehead and roll the head a very small amount to the left. Apply the fingers of your right hand on the right side of the neck gently, on or underneath the lateral processes of the cervical vertebrae. Press these vertebrae to the left so that the head is brought back to the "nose-up" position, even if the place of support from underneath has not changed. Release the pressure of your right fingers slightly without taking them away, and allow the head and neck to return elastically to the starting position. Repeat until you find the optimal place, direction, and amount of pressure to use, and until the movement establishes itself as feasible. That is the relative conjugate movement for the rolling (rotation) of the head to the right. If this feels appropriate and seems harmless (for the pupil), then try similar manipulons for other movements of the head, such as lateral bending of the neck and extension of the neck.

5. Touch Supplementing the Kinesthetic Sense

Patterns of action that are "low-level" controlled usually have afferent (sensory) impulses—proprioceptive or other—that do not reach the "upper-level" sensory brain segments. The person is, in other words, unaware of certain details concerning that action. This situation serves a good biological purpose, that is, it saves us from having to be distracted by a continuous flow of irrelevant and useless information about patterns of action that are performed automatically.

If, on the contrary, the pattern of action has to be adapted or changed, then some of these afferent impulses need to be brought up into the higher sensory centers. The teacher can, by *touching* the relevant participating body parts, supply sensory information about what these parts are doing. In this way, additional parts of the pupil's proprioceptive information flow come into the pupil's awareness and become thus "high-level" controlled.

An example: With the pupil lying on one side (head supported, thighs flexed), push the spine from the neck towards the pelvis by applying one hand to the shoulder near the neck and release in a rhythmic way (this manipulon has been previously described). The pelvis will rock somewhat. Continue the movement with one hand, while placing the other on the pelvis from above (a conforming manipulon). This will draw the pupil's attention to the fact that the pelvis is moving and in this way the quality of that movement will improve.

Or, have the pupil lying on the back. Take one of the arms by grasping it at the elbow and hold it so that the upper arm is vertical. Lift it slightly and let it come down. Continue to do this with one of your hands, while with the other you touch the shoulderblade from underneath, so that this hand moves together with the shoulderblade. If the pupil was resisting the participation of the shoulderblade before, he may now engage it more readily.

While making this last movement with the arm, observe the pupil's head. In some cases it might roll to the side, as if shoulder and neck are one rigid piece. Continue to produce the movement with one hand, while using the other hand to touch the head from the opposite side, as a confining manipulon. It might be enough, for example, merely to touch the ear with the back of your hand. This will bring to the pupil's attention the fact that an extra component has been involuntarily added by him to the movement initiated by you. The movement of the shoulder may now be differentiated from the head movement. This constitutes in itself a newly learned pattern.

Supplementing the kinesthetic sense by touching may be useful in relation to the *muscles* involved in the carrying out of a pattern. When a muscle is used unsatisfactorily (it may be spastic, too strong, too weak, jerky, or used superfluously), then the afferent (sensory) impulses coming from that muscle are, obviously, established components of that pattern. The teacher can try to produce such a pattern (by a conforming or leading manipulon) and *simultaneously* touch or palpate the involved muscle. The simultaneousness of the palpation and the movement creates a way for the pupil to associate them and to perceive them as parts of the same pattern. This may, accordingly, change the pattern in the pupil's representation and enable him to envisage the voluntary implementation of such a change. The palpation can be done by sliding the hand over the muscle either lengthwise or across, but sometimes a steady pressure over the muscle's belly—while the movement is being done by the other hand—will do. Any of these handlings should be gentle, just enough to be perceived as dealing with the muscle rather than the skin or the underlying layer of fat.

Sometimes the same hand can serve to produce both actions. An example: With the pupil on the stomach, sit facing the right side and put both your palms, parallel to each other, flat over the right-side extensors of the pupil's back. Push with your palms slightly, aiming the bases of the hands and the thumbs towards each other. In this way, you will produce a side bend of the spine (the convexity to the left), simultaneously shortening the muscle that is supposed to participate in this movement when it is produced by the pupil. You can produce the same movement in several different ways; for example, by pushing slightly with your left hand the right side of the pelvis towards the head, while dealing with the respective muscle (the right-side extensor of the back) with your right hand.

Another way of varying the approach is to do as described above and, instead of letting the pelvis come back immediately, hold it there steadily for some seconds (a confining manipulon), until you feel the impulse to return it, as when the pupil begins to inhale. The coming-back could be used as a first stage in continuing into the opposite movement (in this example, a bend of the spine with the convexity to the right). The leading manipulon could then be, for example, to gently pull the pupil's spine toward you by hooking the spinous processes of a few vertebrae with the fingertips of both your hands while simultaneously sliding both your thumbs away from each other over the same muscle (which now becomes an antagonist), so that its lengthening becomes more clearly associated with this movement.

There is of course the third possibility of a muscle needing attention for reasons other than being an agonist or antagonist in some unsatisfactory way, namely being a "parasitic synergist" (see p. 46). The same approach as with an interfering antagonist is then appropriate.

In closing, it should be said that "working" on muscles without simultaneously making clear the link with corresponding movement patterns has questionable teaching value. It might even disrupt the pupil's kinesthetic attention, which has already been successfully brought forth by the teacher. Nevertheless, certain exploratory manipulons may necessarily have this "handling-muscles-only" quality.

6. Effort Substitution

Lengthening or stretching a muscle by an agent outside the organism will elicit, as a reflex response, an increased activation of that muscle in opposition to this lengthening. This is the well-known stretch reflex, by which afferent stimuli coming from the stretch-receptors situated in the muscle have an excitatory effect on the respective motor neurons in the spinal cord. The main biological functions of this mechanism are to maintain a steady muscular tonus and to activate antigravitational muscles needed to move and to act in the gravitational field. It is a self-regulatory feedback mechanism which, most of the time, does not need voluntary attention. Yet, in certain situations, voluntary (high-level) control can of course inhibit that reflex, such as when I decide to let my arm fall down after support has suddenly been taken away from beneath. I am recalibrating, for that moment at least, the scale of values for evaluating the relevant proprioceptive input, so that, rather than immediately contracting the arm to prevent its fall, I inhibit this reflex. The increase in muscular tonus that should have been elicited by the stretch reflex is reduced or even temporarily abolished. Such a recalibration is probably going on, continuously or intermittently, mainly in relation to refined, highly differentiated patterns of action.

In patterns less amenable to high-level control, as in movements of the trunk, for example, this voluntary recalibration is less frequent. It happens during strong efforts, for example, that the muscle's tone increases uncontrollably, as in some cases of sudden "low back pain." In cybernetic parlance, the feedback loop of the stretch reflex has its "gain" too high, and there is no agent from outside the loop to recalibrate it. A change in the "higher-order feedforward" is called for (see chapter 2). This situation might become even more pronounced when there is an impairment of cerebral control over the motor system.

A manipulon that brings the ends of an overtense muscle

nearer to one another, maintaining the shortened distance (a confining manipulon) for ten to twenty seconds, can modify the sensory pattern produced by both the muscle's length-receptors and tension-receptors. The flow of excitatory impulses coming to the respective motor neurons in the spinal cord becomes diminished. Moreover, since the antagonist muscle is slightly stretched, it will, after the release, contract and possibly inhibit the agonist. The latter, in other words, will soften and become lengthened. Reciprocal inhibition will gradually re-establish itself in this pair of antagonists. Such a manipulon should be gentle and not forced. The degree to which one brings the "insertion" and "origin" of the muscle nearer to each other should be small, especially when there is pain involved. A few repetitions of the manipulon, combined perhaps with other approaches to elucidate the situation, will bring this into the pupil's awareness, and help change (recalibrate) the motor response to proprioceptive stimuli.

One example of this sort of confining manipulon was given in chapter 3; three others follow. In the case of taut pectoral muscles: The pupil lies on the back, knees drawn up so that the legs are as in standing, feet shoulder-wide apart. The teacher lifts one shoulderblade from underneath slightly, away from the underlying surface, so that it slides a little bit relative to the chest, without moving the chest itself. It is held there and then released. The movement is repeated until the shoulder drops down easily. A juxtaposing manipulon, comparing this shoulder with the other one, may shortcut the way to resolve the tension on the other side.

In the case of taut abdominal muscles: With the pupil in the position just described, both shoulderblades are lifted simultaneously, this time until the small ribs begin to approach the pelvis. The position is held there. Having substituted outside effort for the effort of the abdominal muscles, they become released and consequently you may see the beginning of a deep inhalation, evoked by the greater freedom gained in the region of the small ribs.

In the case of taut extensors of the back: The pupil lies on the stomach. The teacher puts both the palms flat, one over the sacrum (the part of the pelvis immediately below the small of the back), the other over the thoracic spine. The most appropriate place for the latter might be different for different pupils. A very slight pressure to bring the sacrum nearer the ribs, will reduce some of the effort of the extensors of the back. Since these muscles overlie the ribs and, when taut, interfere with the movements of the last two pair of ribs (the "floating ribs"), the release of this tautness can have, as with the previous example, a similar result—a deep inhalation. If this occurs, then a conforming manipulon, a gentle touching of the ribs with flat hands over the back and going in the direction of the inhalation, will enhance the "upper-level" assimilation of this pattern.

7. Breathing

Breathing as a movement pattern has already been mentioned. It is an important and complex function that affects a number of other functions. Moreover, this influence is reciprocal. Without embarking on a full discussion of breathing, we should make a few remarks from the point of view of Functional Integration.

The primary purpose of breathing is of course to supply the lungs with the oxygen needed in the blood and to eliminate the carbon dioxide brought by the bloodstream back to the lungs. The rate of metabolism and, with it, the uptake of oxygen, and the production of carbon dioxide depend on muscular exertion as a foremost factor.

The uptake of oxygen during continuous and vigorous muscular effort may increase to about twenty times the uptake at the resting level. The respiratory apparatus is *able to adjust* itself within quite wide limits. This adjustment is produced mainly by changing the volume of air exchanged with each breathing cycle, or by changing the frequency of these cycles, or by changing both these parameters at the same time. There are, nevertheless, a few additional parameters that can change as a way of adjusting the breathing functions to changing needs and circumstances.

The adaptability of the respiratory apparatus comes into play for reasons other than respiration. We use the incoming air flow for smelling. The outgoing air is used for voice production (as in crying, laughing, talking, singing, or playing a wind instrument, for example), as well as for coughing, sneezing, or any expulsive effort, such as voluntarily blowing air at something.

Curiously enough, this quite complex function of the breathing apparatus, with its inherent adaptability, does not acquire its *basic pattern* through learning. The pattern is *hereditary*. Anyone breathes within seconds after birth and "knows" how to cough, to yawn, or to sneeze.

This phylogenetically learned pattern is very old and deeply "wired-in"; indeed, it is quite similar for most vertebrates. Nevertheless, anyone can *voluntarily change* the rhythm or the quantity of breathing, at least for limited periods. Moreover, various motor patterns, by using muscles also involved in respiration, can influence or be influenced by respiration. For example, any strong activation of the flexor muscles of the trunk will interfere with breathing. Try lying on the floor on your back while lifting the extended legs off the floor, so that the heels are five centimeters away from the floor. The interference with breathing will become clear at once. Also remember that a motor pattern such as a strong activation of the flexors might be part of an emotional syndrome, such as anxiety. (See *Body and Mature Behavior.*)

Improving one's breathing can often be an important, even necessary task. On the other hand, any facilitation of the breathing process is only a reminder to the system of something that has already been there a long time. You do not learn to breathe; you can only learn how to interfere less with this well-established pattern, so that it may adapt itself more easily to various circumstances in the environment and to the biological necessities of one's existence.

It is clear from the foregoing that different levels of control are involved in the various functions of the breathing apparatus and that the basic breathing pattern can be renewed or restored if needed by clarifying it in connection with patterns of higher-level control. Conversely, any improvement of the breathing pattern will raise the quality of related functions.

In dealing with the motor components of the respiratory mechanism, one has to consider the two main areas: *(a)* the movements of the diaphragm and *(b)* the movements of the rib cage.

The diaphragm muscle separates the abdominal organs from those contained in the chest. It is a vault-like muscle, with its dome directed upwards. Its fibers run more or less radially and are attached to the lower circumference of the thoracic cage from the inside. By contracting, these fibers pull the central part of the muscle (the central tendon) down, so that the volume of the lungs is increased. This happens during inspiration. The lowering of the diaphragm pushes the abdominal organs downwards, so that the abdomen protrudes slightly. The external intercostal muscles, being activated synergistically, lift the ribs, so that the volume of the chest increases still more by widening transversally. The ribs also move at the point of their articulations with the respective vertebrae and the sternum. Each pair of ribs forms a surface that slants down, mainly forward, and somewhat to the sides. The above-mentioned rib movement that occurs in inspiration elevates the ribs, so that the slanting decreases, the ribs flare out to the sides, and the sternum rises, moving away from the spine. As for the diaphragm, its combined movement within the rib cage could be briefly described as a lowering of the dome with a lifting and widening of its circumference.

In expiration, the diaphragm relaxes. The elastic recoil of the thoracic and abdominal walls, assisted by the internal intercostal muscles and sometimes additionally by the abdominal muscles, brings the ribs down and the dome of the diaphragm up. This decreases the volume of the lungs and air is pushed out.

The amount of involvement of different muscles in producing the respiratory movements, or in interfering with them, is subject to many variations. There is, therefore, purely from a motor point of view, a great variety in the quality of breathing movements. This can be found during the varied activity of the same person, as well as among different individuals. In addition, there is the quantitative variability related to frequency and amount of air exchange already mentioned.

There are a surprisingly large number of circumstances that can interfere with the adjustability of the breathing function. An important instance is the *body pattern of anxiety,* which Feldenkrais describes (*Body and Mature Behavior,* p. 83 ff.) as an instinctive, inborn contraction of the flexor muscles simultaneous with an inhibition of the extensors (antigravity muscles). This is a reaction to the sensation of imminent danger, in the case of being attacked, for example, or when there is fear of falling or losing the ground underfoot.

A violent stimulation of the vestibular apparatus (which is concerned with sensing acceleration of movement and eliciting related adaptive motor reflexes), or a sudden, loud noise will usually provoke that pattern of reacting to the fear of falling. "This pattern of flexor contraction is reinstated every time the individual reverts to passive protection of himself when lacking the means, or doubting his power, of active resistance. The extensors or antigravity muscles are perforce partially inhibited" (ibid., p. 92). Moreover, this pattern may in many instances persist, thus becoming a low-level controlled habit, long after the anxiety-producing agent has disappeared.

Besides the anxiety complex, there are other processes that produce a rigid muscular connection between the pelvis and the thorax, thus diminishing the adaptability of the breathing apparatus.

For example, A. S., a woman of twenty-six, showed a slight scoliosis (lateral curvature of the vertebral column), with the convexity to the left in her lumbar spine and some difficulties in breathing. It turned out that she had had an appendectomy three years before, and she still felt the need to protect the scar, which she believed was a "weak spot." When, through Functional Integration, she experienced the possibility of letting her right-side ribs participate in breathing, not only were her abdominal muscles (the scar included) relieved from a constant stress, but also her scoliosis disappeared, proving that it had been produced by this unilateral muscular contraction.

S. D., a woman of forty-six, while becoming aware of a breathing pattern that involved the movement of her ribs more than her usual, habitual pattern, remarked, "You know, I have had difficulties in breathing for many years. I even know when it started." I said, "Wasn't it from the age of twelve?" She said, "Exactly! I was concerned that my breasts were becoming too prominent, and what I did was to tuck in my belly. Now I don't mind, and since now I see the connection, I know how to deal with the habit."

A short list of manipulons related to the working of the respiratory apparatus follows. Each of these manipulons stimulates or facilitates one component of the complex pattern of breathing. If used sporadically, they will not necessarily affect breathing, but if used as integrating manipulons (after prior preparation using related patterns), they will likely produce results. There is no attempt here to change an existing pattern of rigid connection between pelvis and thorax, but rather to produce a situation in which the pupil's system may positively respond in a way already "known" to him.

The pupil lies on the left side, knees and hip joints flexed comfortably, with some support underneath the head. Sitting behind the pupil's back, the teacher finds the area of the vertebral column nearest to the ground and at that point supports a few neighboring vertebrae (two or more) with the fingers (using both hands) from underneath their spinous processes, as if attempting to straighten out the column parallel to the ground. Proceeding from an exploratory manipulon through a gentle leading one (working with the breathing in) to a confining manipulon, the teacher supports the column steadily. If the need is felt, only the right hand is left supporting the column while the left palm is placed flat on the pupil's right shoulder-blade, leading it gently into abduction, as if helping the pupil to "reach out" with the right elbow in front of the face. This adds a slight twist to the spine and leaves the head extended and the right-side ribs free to flare out.

The pupil lies on the left side, as before. By slightly pushing behind the right iliac crest towards the shoulder (confining manipulon), the teacher reduces the effort of the abdominal muscles connecting the right lower ribs with that crest. While doing this with the right hand, one supports the vertebral column (as before) with the left hand, so that the angle between the column and the right-side pelvis is diminished somewhat (fig. 10). Cease pushing the pelvis as soon as an inhalation begins, but still leave the hands in place (conforming manipulon). Start again with the next movement of exhalation.

The pupil lies on one side. With both hands on the shoulder joint and scapula respectively and, with the most minute pressure possible, slowly slide the scapula very slightly in various directions over the rib cage (exploring and conforming manipu-

Fig. 10

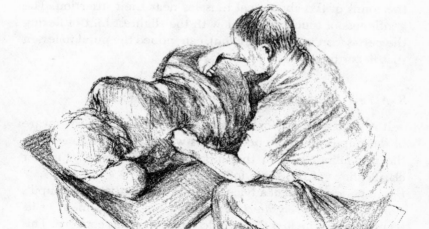

lons alternating with leading ones). Eventually, the pupil will find how to decrease the muscular connection between the rib cage and the moving parts, so that the scapula will "float" and the ribs will then be free to flare out.

The pupil lies on the stomach, the face to the left, the left knee bent and drawn forward, so that the pelvis is elevated on its left side. The right arm rests alongside the body and the left arm is bent, so that the elbow is somewhere in front of the face. The teacher sits facing the pupil's left arm and takes the pupil's left shoulder joint with both hands, the fingers supporting it from underneath and the thumbs touching from above. Making the smallest possible movements, the teacher helps the pupil find a way to have the shoulder "floating." The position is held that way for a moment or so, until the pattern is established as both possible and comfortable.

The pupil lies on the back, the knees drawn up with the feet placed on the bench, slightly apart. The teacher touches the two prominent frontal ridges of the pelvic bone on both sides of the lower abdomen (the anterior superior iliac spine). The hands are flat, as if intending to flex the pelvis, bringing these two points nearer to the chest (fig. 11). In doing this one senses the tonus of the abdominal muscles near their insertion. The gentleness of touch, together with the slightest hint of flexing the pelvis (confining manipulon), can induce the pupil to lessen that flexor tonus.

8. A Few Additional Remarks on Levels of Control

It is good practice for the teacher to be continuously aware of the pupil's level of control. This will enable him to address the prevailing level in the appropriate "language." Further clarifications of this topic follow.

As a general word of advice it should be said that if the pupil's system is excessively *alert* to any possible infringement of its security, then the first thing to do is to lessen this concern. This can be done, for example, by shifting or directing the pupil's

Fig. 11

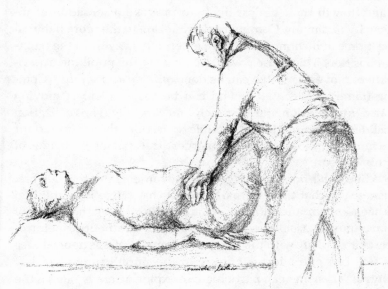

interest to some area of action evoking security, comfort, and successful functioning.

It has already been pointed out that there can be an *overaction of the flexors* when there is a state of *regression,* whatever may be the process that produced this regression. Since acting directly against the flexors is not advisable, one could perform a *nondifferentiated* movement that does not require participation of a tense flexor. Then one could gradually shift over to a *differentiated* movement, where the easy participation of that flexor would be more readily allowed. A way of envisaging this process is the following: the protective pattern involving this flexor is left unaroused, while the flexor is rendered free to function as an antagonist to the appropriate extensor. This latter will occur in the framework of the mechanism of reciprocal inhibition, which earlier might have been interfered with.

Any movement of extension away from the middle of the

body should be done slowly, especially during the exploratory stage. It will then be less likely to provoke a sensation of insecurity or danger. Coming back by flexion to the more habitual position can be done faster than extension away from the habitual position. This is also a way to convey to the pupil the experience of movements that can be done *quickly and safely.* "Coming home" is always safe and can be done quickly; "moving away" must be done rather slowly and carefully. The realization that fast movements are feasible is frequently an important learning experience that enlarges the person's image of achievement.

While *exploring the range* of a movement, the teacher first makes sure that the habitual sector of that range is established as well-known and familiar. This middle part of the range of movement is usually somewhere around the neutral point of least effort. Only with the acknowledgement of this neutral area as safe can one address oneself to the pupil's upper level of control. Then one can participate in exploring areas "across the border."

An extension movement that is "new" to the pupil is preferably preceded by a corresponding flexion, even if there is no question of danger. By a repetitive alternation of flexion and extension it is possible to provide the pupil with the feeling of security associated with flexion (or nonextension) by putting the *emphasis* on flexion. This may be done by pausing for a moment at the end of each flexion and producing an extension as if it were only to prepare for the next flexion. This emphasis on one direction can, of course, be later shifted to the other one, but not before the teacher feels that the image of the whole pattern has been clarified.

As an example of such a procedure, one of the ways of clarifying the overactivity of a tense pectoral muscle is as follows: The pupil lies on his back. The teacher takes the pupil's right hand and places it on the pupil's left shoulder (or somewhere nearby), so that the elbow lies on the chest. With his left hand the teacher lightly pushes the elbow into the chest to emphasize the nonextension, while using his other hand to support the right scapula from underneath. This movement is repeated, alternating it with an imperceptible lifting of the elbow from the chest. The emphasis is still on the flexion of the shoulder joint. The moment comes when the teacher feels that the outside effort has substituted for the effort of the pupil's pectoral muscle. The emphasis can be changed gradually towards a slight extension of the arm as the auxiliary movement of supporting the scapula continues, first in phase with the flexion, then in phase with the extension. Eventually, the elbow will come up easily as the upper arm extends diagonally over the head.

Here is one more example. To hyperextend the neck while moving the chin away from the chest is felt by many people as dangerous or even impossible (we are not speaking of a situation where there is structural damage of any kind). The pupil lies supine. The teacher holds the pupil's head by supporting it from underneath with one hand at a comfortable height. With his other hand he moves the pupil's chin slightly down, as if "looking at the navel." As this flexion is repeated the teacher might increase the efficiency of the action by suggesting to the pupil to look up and down, following the movements of his head. The linkage of the eye movements with the neck movements thus helps in the process of clarification. The eye-neck linkage is, of course, low-level controlled. In doing this, the teacher has the advantage of establishing a new or renewed pattern by using a way of functioning that is already well ingrained in the CNS.

These examples are not meant to imply that extension must be achieved at all costs. It is important, however, to provide the pupil with the insight that it is not necessary to act continuously against extension. In other words, the pupil should be able to distinguish sensorily, and not only intellectually, between not *choosing* to do a certain movement and *involuntarily* and continuously organizing the body against such a movement. This insight, sensorily established, can be most helpful in getting rid of certain superfluous avoidance patterns.

If the pupil's CNS is reasonably calm and not alerted to possible danger, then even *"risky patterns"* can be tried out. The pupil's self-image can thus be supplemented and broadened. The pupil might then be better equipped to adjust to situations ordinarily occurring in everyday life in which it would not be possible to rely solely on well-established patterns of action. A pattern of movement that is new or surprising without being dangerous in itself might be perceived by the pupil as risky and should be approached with due preparation. Sometimes, of course, the risk is quite real, as when it is related to the pupil's structural limitations.

Suppose that a clarification of the movement patterns of the forearm (pronation and supination), wrist, and fingers is called for, and that the intention is to create a different pattern from the habitual. One of the ways of doing this is to have the pupil lie on the stomach, face turned to the left, and the right arm alongside the body. The right elbow is then slightly lifted, so that the back of the hand can be easily placed on the pelvis, or even higher up on the back (fig. 12). This position might be perceived as unsafe, since it is quite removed from the habitual. If needed, an appropriate preparation for this position can be achieved by the movements of the shoulder and shoulder-blade. On the other hand, the firm contact of the pupil's forearm with the back, insured by the teacher's touch during the subsequent stages of manipulation, will remove much of the sensation of riskiness and instill more confidence and cooperation.

It is often a good practice to begin working *with the better side*. For example, if there is a "problem" (pain or impairment) on one side, right or left, then one can clarify first the "good" side, familiarizing oneself as well as the pupil with the muscular tonus and ranges of movement on the side where the alertness to change and danger are *less* pronounced. When the same proceedings are carried out, perhaps to a lesser extent, on the "worse" side, the program is then *already* known beforehand

Fig. 12

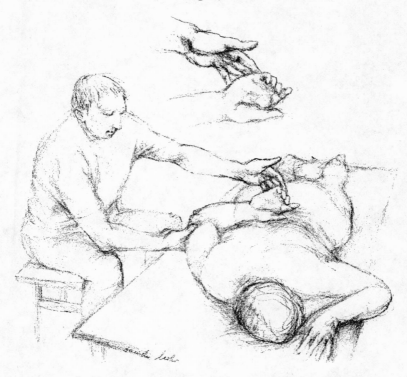

and the pupil knows what to anticipate. The way is then free for juxtaposing the situations on either side, as well as for shifting learned skills from one side of the body—and brain—to the other.

Part III

FURTHER TECHNICAL
CONSIDERATIONS

6. Some Physical Principles Involved in Functional Integration

I wish now to explain some of the physical concepts and principles used in describing and analyzing movements of the human body. These concepts are important in understanding the physical aspects of motor functioning as well as certain technical aspects of the various manipulations. This understanding will enable the teacher to increase both his efficiency and the clarity of the information flow involved in the pupil-teacher interaction. Along with this discussion of physical principles, examples of manipulons will be given in which the use of these principles is particularly apparent. The reader should not consider this a chapter in physics so much as a way of pointing out certain basic facts.

Let us take the concepts of *force* and *pressure*, for example, as they appear in what is called classical mechanics. Force acting on a body involves the acceleration (or deceleration) of that body, its deformation, or both—acceleration being the rate of change of the body's velocity. The exact formulation of these relationships is found in Newton's Laws and the law of deformation as it relates to elastic bodies.

If two bodies act upon one another by direct contact, then both undergo corresponding accelerations (or decelerations), as well as elastic deformations, through forces of *equal magnitude* that are *opposed* in their directions. This is Newton's Third Law. The accelerations will be in inverse relation to the masses of the bodies, that is, the larger the mass, the smaller its acceleration (Newton's Second Law). The kind of forces encountered in this work, apart from muscular forces, are elastic forces (forces related to elastic deformation), gravitational forces, and frictional forces.

Pressure is the amount of force per unit of area, expressed, for example, in kilograms per square centimeter or pounds per square inch. Pressure is what happens in terms of local impact when two bodies are in close contact. If the force involved in this contact is transmitted to a larger area, then the pressure is proportionately smaller, and vice versa. This fact is, of course, decisive for what is happening locally at the point of pressure. It explains why a sharp knife, for example, penetrates more easily than a blunted one; the surface where the force is applied is small, hence the pressure is proportionately very great. The area of the ski is many times greater than that of the sole of the shoe and thus the ski is prevented from sinking into the snow. A padded surface is more comfortable to lie upon, simply because the increased area of contact makes the local pressure smaller.

This last remark reveals something of obvious importance in the practice of making the pupil feel more comfortable and ready for a learning experience. The force used by the teacher in manipulations, small as it may already be, will be felt to be more pleasant and less intrusive if applied on a larger surface with the flat of the teacher's hand, rather than with the fingertips.

Pressure applied to an area is a force acting at right angles to the surface of contact. The role of *friction* becomes apparent when we consider two bodies pressed against one another by a force that is at an angle different from a right angle. In this instance a *sliding* movement of one body relative to the other will result, unless there is enough frictional force to prevent this sliding. The diagonal force in such a case is said to consist of two components related to two actions: one is the pressure itself, acting at right angles to the surface; the other is the production of the above-mentioned sliding, unless it is counteracted by friction. The maximum amount of frictional force that will prevent the sliding is in itself dependent on the pressure: the greater the pressure, the greater the friction. Apart from this, frictional forces also depend on the particular materials of the two bodies.

If the acting force is directed at right angles to the surface, then there is no friction. It is a well-known fact that standing on a very slippery surface is possible only if the surface is horizontal, since the force of gravity producing the pressure is then at right angles to the surface. We are able to stand on an inclined surface only because friction is present. Moreover, our ability to accelerate (or decelerate) is made possible in most instances because of friction: we can begin to move forward or stop on a horizontal surface by using the existing friction.

These facts are so basic in everyday life that little attention is paid to them. Only when friction fails are we caught by surprise and forced to rely on fast-acting reflexes, as when stepping inadvertently on a slippery surface.

Lubrication is a way of considerably decreasing frictional forces and is used when one wants easy movement to be possible. On the other hand, increased friction is needed for braking, stopping, or preventing movement. To enhance friction, special materials are chosen. However, the crucial factor determining friction is, as has already been pointed out, the amount of pressure that pushes bodies against one another. A wet glass held between our fingers might slide away, but by increasing the pressure of our fingers we increase the frictional force and stop the sliding.

Wear and tear caused by friction and the *heating up* of moving bodies when friction is present are well-known phenomena —simply think of the action of striking a match. Friction inside or on the human body can be destructive as well. All the joints used in movements have some kind of lubrication that ordinarily works quite satisfactorily. Nevertheless, friction in the joints can increase and become destructive, not only if that lubrication fails, but also if the bones are pushed forcefully against one another, either by excessive muscular action or by some violent manipulation.

Any handling that is not directed at right angles to the surface of touch obviously, then, involves friction between the teacher's hand and the pupil's skin (or clothing). Sometimes this is done deliberately, as when exploring the location of a skeletal detail by sliding the skin over a bone, or when exploring the texture of a tense muscle. In this case, it should be done in the gentlest manner. Otherwise, sliding should be avoided. The teacher always uses, when possible, any protruding parts of a bone, such the bones' processes or condyles, as "stops" to prevent the sliding of the hand.

Force can be transmitted through the pupil's body in a variety of ways, for example, by pressing from the head towards the pelvis or from the feet towards the head. In order to achieve an efficient transmission through the skeleton, this pressure should propagate *at right angles* to the surfaces of the respective joints. This requirement is especially important when it relates to the vertebrae, or more specifically to the transversal facets of the bodies of the vertebrae. If this is not done, there will be a component of the force parallel to the surfaces of contact between the adjacent bones, which will tend to produce a transverse sliding effect called "shearing stress." This can be damaging to the structure and, even when done very gently, it will be uncomfortable to the pupil.

Shearing stress should be avoided by the teacher. Of course, the teacher is not supposed to gauge exact angles each time; the issue is not purely a geometrical one. It should rather be appreciated sensorily and also in terms of the body functions involved. If one starts with the slightest push, looking for the direction that will allow the farthest transmission of this push, then it should not provoke a defensive reaction from the pupil.

Increased friction in a joint is sometimes related to arthritic changes that have occurred in this joint. Diminishing the pressure between the two bones can decrease the friction and alleviate discomfort or pain in case it is related to overacting muscles.

It is well known that from the mechanical point of view parts of the skeleton act as *levers*. Many bones can be considered pivoted at one place, while two forces act on them in two different places that are at a certain distance from the pivot. In other words, they act as levers. Let's take the example of the foot: When one lifts oneself up on the toes, the foot is pivoted on the floor at the base of the toes, and two forces act on it: (1) the taut calf muscles that pull vertically up through the Achilles tendon attached to the heel, and (2) the force of gravity (the weight of the body, or part of it) that pushes down vertically, through the leg bones to the ankle joint. Yet, the same foot can be considered a lever in other ways, when it is performing different functions.

In a sitting position, when one pushes something away with the toes, the same muscles are acting at the heel, but the foot is pivoted at the ankle joint and the pushed object presses back at the toes.

Another interesting example is the head, when it is in an upright position. The skull is pivoted at the uppermost vertebra. The center of gravity of the head is located in front of the pivot. Thus, the force of gravity (the weight of the head) acting vertically down through this point, has to be counteracted by the pull of the posterior neck muscles if the head is not to drop forward. This is an example of a group of muscles that have to work habitually and almost continually, even when the body is organized in its most efficient way: This means that a certain tonus is always present in the neck muscles without our conscious attention. The person might not become aware of it, unless, for some reason, it becomes excessive and bothersome. A similar tonus is always present in the muscles that prevent the jaw from dropping down by its weight.

The quantitative way of looking at levers is expressed in a well-known formula that stipulates the condition for a lever's equilibrium: the ratio of the forces equals the inverse ratio of the lever's hands. The lever's "hands" are the distances of the pivot to the straight lines on which the forces are acting. Without having to apply this formula in a numerical way, one nevertheless can be helped by it in understanding certain mechanical features of motor functions, and of efficient manipulations as well.

It is helpful for the teacher to figure out (1) which part of the pupil's body is to be involved in movement, (2) the pivot (if any) as the nonmoving point around which the movement is performed, and (3) the two forces or groups of forces: the teacher's force and the resisting force. The latter could be weight, friction, elastic forces, or the pupil's muscular efforts. In calling them "resisting forces," I do not mean to imply that there should be an attempt to overcome them. The decision whether this will be the case or not can never be taken on mechanical grounds alone.

It might happen that the teacher has no choice but to act near the pivot of some "lever." But, ideally, one should work on a site more distant from the pivot. The acting force will then be smaller and gentler; the movement will be greater and therefore easier to control in terms of its direction and quantity.

The movements of the trunk in flexion and extension can be regarded as a lever action, with the upper half of the trunk being pivoted at the lumbar vertebrae. The forces acting in the direction of flexion are the weight of the upper part of the body from the pivot up and the pull of the abdominal muscles. The extensors of the back act on this "lever" in the opposite direction, that is, in extension. The latter forces have their line of action much nearer to the pivot than the abdominal muscles do. It follows that any increase in the tension of the abdominal muscles calls for an increase in the tension of the back muscles several times the intensity of that of the abdominal muscles, in order to preserve the same posture. It is clear that a small increase in tonus in the abdominal muscles, if done continuously, puts great stress on the back muscles, and thus decreases significantly the mobility of the lumbar spine.

The terms "potential energy" and "kinetic energy" were used earlier when we were dealing with antigravitational patterns and the efficient use of the skeleton (chapter 5). Once again it should be mentioned that the state of *highest potential energy* is tantamount to instability, but that at the same time, this instability provides a starting point for movement without preliminary preparation. Seen in this light, the upright stance is a good starting point for action and movement. Walking (at least on a horizontal surface) and running are a continuous losing and recovering of balance and, if there is very little lowering and raising of the center of gravity, the main energy expenditure ("work" in the mechanical sense) is against friction. This is most easily accomplished if the potential energy can be kept at its highest.

In mechanical terms, work done by muscular effort produces either kinetic energy (movement) or heat (by friction and deformation). The latter possibility, when produced in the body, is harmful and destructive. Pushing hard at a wall or banging it with one's fist will not change the wall much, but it will damage the fist. The mechanical viewpoint thus allows a *criterion for efficiency*, applied to a person's neuro-motor functioning. Muscular work that produces more movement and less heat can be considered more efficient, yet this is a very fragmentary way of looking at human efficiency, since it leaves out considerations of quality.

On the other hand, providing a person with the sensory experience that less than the habitual muscular effort is needed to keep the posture at ease and efficient is in itself invaluable. It means using muscles only when needed or wanted, instead of maintaining unnecessary muscular tonus.

The concept of *elasticity* is usually confused by the everyday notion that elastic bodies are those that have their form easily changed and then revert back to the same shape immediately after the action of the distorting forces ceases, such as various springs, rubber, and other flexible materials, or a quantity of gaseous material confined under pressure, such as a balloon or a playing ball. In fact, up to a certain degree of deformation that depends on the body's physical properties, all bodies are elastic. If the limit of elasticity is overstepped (if the deformation produced by some force is more than this certain amount), the change is no longer reversible. We might not be aware of it, but by putting a finger on the surface of a table, or on any rigid object, we deform that table to a minute extent, and the resistance we feel, small or large, is precisely the elastic force that comes with the deformation. Within the limits of elasticity (when not overstepping the above-mentioned limit), the amount of deformation is proportional to the magnitude of the force producing it.

The force needed to produce a similar deformation is different for different bodies. Moreover, differences relating to the limit of elasticity for various bodies and materials can be quite considerable. Compare, for example, the change in the length of a rubber band, the gradually growing force needed to produce this elongation, and the limit beyond which it will break, with a similar experiment done with a piece of yarn. Compare, as well, the bending of a piece of cardboard until it folds, with the bending of a sheet of glass until it breaks.

In Functional Integration we find elasticity or "quasi-elasticity" related to the pupil's body in different ways. It goes without saying that we don't consider going near these limits as they were mentioned in the last paragraph. We often find that in doing a manipulation we encounter a resistant force which becomes greater, the greater the movement done. Once we let go of the moved part, it returns to its previous place. In other words, we encounter an elastic resistance.

Apart from the inherent elasticity of the various body tissues, there are other circumstances that produce a kind of interaction, as if an elastic force were involved. Appreciation of this distinction can be important for the functional understanding of certain situations. Three of these will be described below.

Suppose an elastic bag filled with water (a hot water bottle) is laid on a flat surface and is pushed from the side. When the pushing stops, it will regain its initial position, not immediately, but after wobbling to and fro a few times. Of course, the movement of the liquid inside the bag adds to the elastic distortion of the bag. A situation somewhat similar to this is occasionally found when pushing slightly on the pupil's body.

A movement made by the teacher might lift the center of gravity of some part of the body (in other words, raise its potential energy). When left alone, this part will return to its initial position by gravity, just as a pendulum that has been pushed away from the vertical position in which it was hanging will return to its original position. Suppose the pupil is lying on the back. A slight push through the extended leg will roll the pelvis into a flexed position in which the pelvis's center of gravity is slightly raised. After the push is relinquished, the pelvis will roll back.

A third possibility is that the return is carried out by the pupil's neuro-motor system on a more or less conscious level. If, in the previous example, the extensors of the back are tense, then the return might be carried out by the stretch reflex after the push has elongated these extensors. It could also have been done on a more conscious level, or even as a voluntary movement. For example, should the sternum be pushed down simultaneous with exhalation, the pupil being supine, expiration may be prolonged. Relinquished at the proper moment, the sternum will then lift itself up again during inspiration, perhaps above the initial position held before pressure was applied. Here we are already far removed from the mere physical elasticity considered earlier, since basic biological functions are now involved.

While doing manipulations, the teacher should have these distinctions in mind. Consider what it would mean if one mistakes the elasticity of the underlying padding or mattress for the "elastic" response of the pupil's body. Under these circumstances, we wouldn't expect much efficiency.

The physical aspect of *repetitive, oscillatory movements* occurring in various manipulons should also be clarified. The purpose of oscillatory movements will be explained further in chapter 7. A simple example, however, such as a pendulum or a see-saw, shows that these movements have in each case their own *"self-regulating frequency."* This frequency, specific in each case, is determined by the distribution of the oscillating body's mass relative to its fixed point or axis, if any, or relative to its position of equilibrium. In the case of a simple pendulum, it is its length: the longer the pendulum, the smaller its frequency. In other words, fewer oscillations will be done during a time unit (such as a minute); the time needed for completing a full to-and-fro movement (a full cycle) is greater. The restoring force, which slows down the pendulum during its movement away from the middle and accelerates it during its return, is a component of the pendulum's weight. Although it is obviously not an elastic force, it still has a mathematical property similar to that of elastic forces, namely, proportionality with the distance from the middle point.

Oscillatory movements do not repeat themselves endlessly. Generally they gradually lose their amplitude, due to friction with surrounding bodies and other factors as well. When this happens, the frequency stays the same. Damped oscillations are bound, in these conditions, to come to a stop ultimately.

An elastic body, or a body upon which elastic forces are acting, can produce oscillatory movements. When a weight, hanging on a helical spring, is pulled down slightly from its point of equilibrium, it will oscillate up and down around this point. A similar thing happens when a taut elastic string is plucked, as in a musical instrument with strings, or when the skin of a drum is struck.

Oscillatory movements may also be described in terms of the transition of potential energy into kinetic energy and vice versa. If it were not for energy loss occasioned by this transition, the movement could last forever. The fact that the oscillations are damped points to the fact that mechanical energy is gradually turned into heat (thermal energy), due to friction and other factors.

If we want the oscillations to go on, as in the case of a swing, we have to add a slight push at the appropriate time; in other words, we must add a small amount of energy to the moving body. The movement can go on in a really regular manner only if the added energy makes up exactly for the losses mentioned before, being neither more nor less than those losses.

It now becomes clear that, through small manipulations of just the right frequency and intensity, we can build up a visible oscillatory movement and sustain it at will. The timing is of course set by the self-regulating frequency of the oscillating body (or part of the body). Again, this special frequency is determined by the mass of the oscillating part and by the manner in which this mass is distributed around the center of oscillation.

Here are a few examples. The pupil lies on the back and the teacher sits facing the legs. A small push at the knee, applied as if with the intention to roll the leg, will bring the entire leg into an inward rotation. After this push is relinquished, the leg will return more or less to its previous position. This may be considered as one complete cycle. Without allowing a rest, the next cycle is initiated by pushing again. If all this is done gently enough, the entire leg is brought into an oscillatory rotation around an axis that extends from the point of support of the heel straight to the hip joint. If one pushes at inappropriate times, either earlier or later than needed, it brings the leg either into forced oscillations with a frequency different from its own, or stops the movement altogether.

Sometimes there is a specific reason that one has difficulty in finding this natural, individual frequency. The pupil may interfere with the oscillations by helping or damping. If the teacher produces a much smaller movement than before, the pupil may recognize his own reaction as disproportionate to what is expected to happen and stop the interference. If this occurs, there has been an increase in the level of control involved.

A second example: The pupil lies on his back with the legs extended. The teacher pushes the pupil's leg from the sole of the foot in the direction of the opposite shoulder or the head.

The oscillating part will, of course, be the pelvis. This can usually be done without much difficulty. Comparing this example with the previous one, we may find that the frequency of the oscillation of the pelvis is significantly smaller than that of the leg in its rotational movement around its axis. There might be a damping action by the abdominal muscles, which decrease the mobility of the connection between the pelvis and the thorax. Eventually this connection might become more flexible and, as the oscillations become easier, the pupil may sense the change in muscular tonus associated with the greater ease of movement.

The teacher will sense this change immediately, because a change in the damping forces will require a smaller amount of pushing to sustain the movement.

Appropriate oscillations of the head may also occur during the previous example. Alternate pushing and pulling through the vertebral column may cause the head to oscillate as well, depending on the tonus of the muscles connecting the head with the thorax and on any change that might have occurred in this tonus. In this case, the teacher will probably have to adjust the frequency of the oscillations.

The reader should now see that physical principles of this kind can be important for our work. In any case, such knowledge is left in the background of one's attention, since it doesn't constitute the main point of Functional Integration. It concerns more the technical aspect of the work and should be an auxiliary resource for the teacher, helping to adapt the teaching skills to various situations.

7. Increasing Efficiency: Directions of Movement, Timing, and the Teacher's Own Body Awareness

In a purely physical sense, efficiency is obviously a desirable goal in producing movement and doing work. Yet the main concern in Functional Integration is the efficiency of the pupil's learning process and the transmission of sensory information. We will elaborate a bit on some of the factors related to this.

The direction of movements occurring in various manipulons should, at least in the beginning, be done in what are called the "cardinal directions." These are "up" and "down," "left" and "right," and "forward" and "backward." We are not using the term "cardinal directions" in the sense of the direction of movement produced by a single muscle or muscle group—a movement produced by a single muscle is "simple" in a certain sense, but might at the same time be perceived as complex by the person doing it. The complexity is in the neuro-motor pattern, which includes inhibition of other muscles, sensory feedback, and other factors. We will speak about cardinal directions as they are perceived within a person's sense of spatial orientation.

The directions "up" and "down" are quite clear to us, obviously, because of our constant preoccupation with gravity, whatever our level of consciousness of this preoccupation may be.

"Left" and "right," as concepts of direction, are rooted in the fact that the body is bilaterally symmetrical (although not entirely so, of course). We are ordinarily made aware of left-right distinctions by comparing both sides of our bodies as to differences in structural details and functional differences, such as right-handedness.

"Forward" and "backward" are connected with the concept of advancing towards or receding from a goal, as well as with the division of the surrounding world into two parts: that part surveyed by our eyes and engaging our interest at the moment, or what is in front of us, and all the rest, which is behind us.

A limb that moves in any of these six cardinal directions can do so in two senses: it can move away from the body (extension, abduction), or toward the body (flexion, adduction). It can be assumed that the cardinal directions are known and fundamentally recognized within the pupil's system, perhaps more so than any of their many combinations. Therefore, it will be efficient to begin any clarification of movement patterns, whether they be habitual or new ones yet to be tried out, with these cardinal directions. The next stage would then be to move on to combinations of directions, such as diagonal movements, rotational movements, and so on.

It is often important to isolate a movement, for example, in a particular joint, as a movement-element of a more complex pattern. Difficulty of movement in a joint might be related to some local, structural change in the joint, or to an element of movement pertaining to this joint that has not been used for a long time and is as if forgotten. Whichever the case, a clarification of the functions of the joint is important in broadening the pupil's image of actions depending on these functions.

Clarification might start with an exploration of the particular neuro-muscular avoidance patterns that have been restricting the use of the joint. In the course of this procedure, the teacher discovers which level of control is involved. The various joints are anatomically different, as are the kinds of movements they allow. Knowledge of relevant anatomy is surely necessary for the teacher, but this alone is not sufficient. Beyond this knowledge, exploratory manipulons are needed to find out what the prevailing directions and ranges of movement are. One must always bear in mind that the anatomically possible range of movement is not necessarily identical with the habitual range.

Unraveling the pupil's potential range of movement in an easy, efficient way can be quite an important learning experience. Normally, a movement which nears the limit of one's range of movement is usually accompanied by an anticipation of the effort needed to reach this limit. Otherwise, the limit wouldn't be perceived as a limit at all. Let us suppose that the pupil is not using any more of the movement range than the usual, habitual one. The mere knowledge of still being far away from the new limit that you have helped him discover will then make movement within the restricted range easier. It will have been freed from the anticipation of effort or of restriction that had formerly accompanied it.

We can illustrate this idea in the following way: Suppose a person who has been living in a small room moves into a much larger room. Even though no more space is used by the person in the larger room, the feeling of being far away from the walls makes him move around much more freely than in the smaller room where the walls put actual restraints on movement. Another illustration: In walking, we might not occupy more than a space of ten inches or so in width. But if a board having exactly this same width is placed over a deep hole, walking over it will not be comfortable at all, since we are now cautiously aware of restrictions we don't have in simple walking—the possibility of stepping to one side if the need arises is present in one situation and quite absent in the other.

We can expect that the awareness of increased ranges of movement in various parts of the body will be perceived by the pupil as an achievement. It is useful to supplement this by appropriate juxtaposing manipulons and perhaps even to draw the pupil's attention to these differences and changes verbally. Still, the principle holds that we must not work directly against established anti-patterns.

For example, some movements of extension should be approached with special caution, such as extending the upper arm with the elbow above the head, extending the head so that the chin moves away from the chest, completely extending the hip joint, or extending the knee joint. Sometimes one finds that even the elbow joint, usually quite mobile, is not easily extended.

The feasibility of such extensions is to be first ascertained by gentle explorations. If there is a clear hint of resistance of any kind, extension should be avoided, at least for the time being, and flexion in the opposite direction should be attempted. Support of the joint by appropriate padding may calm the hyperalertness of the pupil's system. A soft support underneath the shoulder below the head or behind the knee joint may often be needed when the pupil is in a supine position. By initiating movements of flexion, the teacher can sense whether the pupil is helping or hampering the movement of coming back from flexion. The hampering indicates that the muscle opposing the extension is working under low-level control. If this changes, the teacher will detect it, and some degree of extension can then be explored. It follows that substituting for the pupil's muscular effort can be efficiently done only if supplemented by the refined sensitivity of the teacher's hands. In the example above, the teacher will have to sense whether the help previously received from the pupil in producing flexion is still being offered or not. If it is, and the return movement from the flexed state (which is actually extension) happens with ease, then the movement is now being controlled at the higher level, and new patterns may be explored.

To clarify the *time factor* in Functional Integration, let us mention three examples of manipulons. First, there is a manipulon that is done just once in temporal isolation, as it were, that serves a definite momentary purpose. Many exploratory manipulons are done in this way, as are positioning manipulons. Even if they are repeated, they are still discrete in character, since no special timing is required. An example of this would be exploring the ease of a certain movement alternately with the palpation of the involved muscle, each manipulon being done once every time.

Any confining manipulon would be another example. The movement is started in one direction and stopped at a certain position. The teacher then waits for a change to be produced by the pupil. This change completes the manipulon. A heightened sensitivity to what is going on in terms of timing is necessary. Sometimes the manipulon will include anticipatory information with regard to timing, such as when the movement done by the teacher is synchronized with the exhalation of the pupil (or the inhalation, as the case might be).

Finally, there are the repetitive manipulons. One kind of repetition, apart from oscillation, is done in order to familiarize the pupil with a new situation or a new pattern of action. The movements can be repeated without pausing, but also without hurry, in order to allow an easy recognition of the pattern or a possible reaction of adaptation or rejection. If the pattern is complex, or if the interference of some other pattern is anticipated, a rest of a few seconds between repetitions should be allowed.

Another kind of repetitive manipulons done with a certain frequency and oscillation, has already been discussed in the previous chapter. It was pointed out that oscillating movements could serve as efficient tools to the teacher. The teacher has to have some sense of rhythm in order to perceive the appropriate frequency of an oscillating body in general, and while working with a pupil in particular. The ability to bring a body into oscillation by applying the smallest possible pushes is dependent upon sensing the natural frequency of that body for a particular kind of oscillation. One may wish to test this on inanimate objects. An automobile, for example, can actually be brought into oscillation by pushing with only one finger, and it will move with a different frequency when rocked from side to side than when rocked up and down.

In order to produce sustained oscillations, the teacher has to oscillate parts of his own body with a prescribed frequency. His body and the pupil's body will then move with the same frequency; in other words, they will be *in resonance,* as it is termed in physics. When this happens, the teacher may easily monitor what is occuring and sense any possible changes in the organization of the pupil's body immediately.

A practical rather than a theoretical understanding of the concept of resonance is needed in order to be able to use this efficiently. Resonance is related to what is usually called "tuning in." The example of pushing a swing into movement is probably the most obvious. Another example is the tuning of a radio set to a certain broadcasting station. Tuning in means bringing both the transmitter and the receiver into resonance, so that both work at the same frequency. The tuning of the receiver is a gradual change in the frequency of electrical oscillations in a certain basic circuit. Only when the frequency is the same as that of the transmitter will the electro-magnetic oscillations produced by the latter influence the oscillations in the receiver. They are then in resonance. The same situation exists, for example, with two strings of a musical instrument or with two different musical instruments. If these two strings operate at the same frequency, then the oscillations (vibrations) of one will bring the other one into oscillation. They are said, accordingly, to be in resonance. The term itself in its more general meaning is actually borrowed from acoustics.

"Tuning in" for the teacher means, first of all, sensing the natural frequency of the oscillating part of the pupil's body and secondly, as already mentioned, letting appropriate parts of the body join in these oscillations. For example, the hand up to the wrist might be used for high frequency movements, and the arm up to the shoulder, or further, including the trunk, for lower frequency movements. Resonance, in the sense outlined before, can be felt sensorily by the teacher as well as by the pupil, as an easy, ongoing oscillation, with both systems engaged in a perfectly joined activity.

The change we might expect in such cases is usually a decrease in the damping forces. If these are merely muscular efforts, then the change is in the improved control the pupil attains over these patterns. From this point of view, oscillatory manipulons simply create one more situation in which neuro-motor learning can take place.

Timing, as related to Functional Integration, has yet another aspect. Repetitive manipulons, with or without oscillation, raise certain questions: *How much? How long?* How much can the pupil's system take? The main concern is that a certain message should come through clearly, but in changing certain ways of acting, the pupil might sometimes be put into a precarious situation. Habitual patterns of action are often a way the system has adapted itself to certain structural restrictions that might have arisen earlier in life. Any change in the way of functioning, where there are structural difficulties, should be approached slowly, if at all. Changes should never deprive the pupil of hard-earned feelings of security, which one obtains only by restricting oneself to what eventually become habitual patterns of action.

To proceed slowly also means to execute movements slowly. Oscillating movements may, in some phases, be quite rapid, and should not be performed at all if slow movements seem to be indicated.

For example, certain structural changes in the cervical verte-brae, such as spondylosis, dictate that any movement of the head or of the neck should be made very slowly, and only small movements—smaller than the pupil himself does—should be considered. In the beginning, no movement should be per-formed directly with the head. Relative conjugate movements with the arms, shoulders, or trunk are to be preferred.

To offer another example, the knee joint might have suffered a tear of some of the ligamental tissue in an accident. If this has not been repaired surgically, which is not always possible, the person will probably use the muscles around the knee in a different way, perhaps with an increased tonus, in order to assure stability and security in the joint. To free this weakened structure from such protective patterns will be destructive and is therefore not to be done. It might happen that this kind of protection is excessive, so that it acts as an exaggerated restriction to movement and is even pain-producing. In this case, the pupil should be helped to reach a higher level of control over his actions in the affected area, thus coming to use the damaged joint in the best possible way.

Examples like this, which indicate the necessity of proceeding cautiously or not at all, are innumerable. On the other hand, if there is no danger in exploring new possibilities, the mere juxtaposition of the changed and the unchanged can be very convincing to the pupil and can also create an awareness of new options of movement.

The foregoing should remind us that the teacher's own body parts are always moving during his manipulations. The CNS is preoccupied with weight, balance, comfort, and other matters, just as it is attentive to and aware of the pupil's preoccupation at this very moment. One should be able to encompass through one's awareness both systems with the same ease.

The criterion of *efficiency* should apply to the teacher's body and its movements in the same manner that it applies to the pupil and to the learning process generally. One should sense how one's own skeleton is being utilized, how the proximal muscles are producing the gross movements, and the distal muscles are being mobilized for gentle touching and sensing. Examples of this are rather obvious. For applying pressure with the hand, the teacher's forearm should be oriented straight along the line of the pressure, so that the appropriate parts of the skeleton will transmit the force. If the teacher is sitting, he can prop his elbow on his knee. The movement of the forearm will be assisted by the pelvis and trunk muscles, removing the otherwise necessary effort of the distal muscles of the hand and the fingers. The fingers will then be free to act as a kind of kinesthetic sense organ, being alert to any minute differences or changes occurring during the manipulation. If this occurs, then both systems, the teacher's and the pupil's, are functioning jointly as one complex system in the neuro-motor realm. The movements are like movements of one complex body, and the sensory communication flows freely in both directions, within this field of mutual interaction, towards both brains. The sensory information arriving at each of the two brains concerns both one's own body as well as the other's. The important part of this is that the pupil gains new information about himself. When this happens we have a learning situation that, one hopes, will be put to good advantage by the teacher.

Part IV

WORKING THROUGH SESSIONS

8. The Form of the Manipulatory Session

After having described in some detail the different manipulations, we should now have a look at these from another point of view. Obviously, the "learning material," or the sensory information perceived by the pupil concerning possible changes in neuro-motor patterns, should be felt to be *adequate, interesting, helpful in solving problems,* and *biologically vital.* Otherwise, these proposed changes might not have enough preponderance to prevail against habitual, ingrained patterns of action. After all, we cannot expect to convince someone to vary motor behavior without providing a feeling that the change is secure, beneficial, satisfying, and needed. There is the possibility that a series of apparently unconnected manipulations will not be understood by the pupil, who might allow them to be performed (if not done too aggressively), and experience them as an accumulation of things happening *at random.* No learning will then take place, hence no reprogramming of the pupil's patterns of action.

For a manipulatory session to engage the *learning process* and to acquire the above-mentioned attributes, the teacher has to structure the content of that session *didactically.* In this way the session becomes a *lesson,* and a series of lessons becomes a course in *neuro-motor tutoring.*

The *didactical approach* to a manipulatory session entails a number of considerations, some touching on principle, some purely practical:

1. The teacher should create a *learning situation* for the pupil, establishing a suitable ambience (sometimes verbally), so that the pupil is ready to participate in the exploration of new patterns of movement. A suitable *starting position* that is most conducive to the pupil's comfort and that takes into consideration any pain or disability should be chosen. This position should also allow some latitude for checking the basic movements of the trunk, head, and limbs.

2. In the course of this checking operation, the teacher should seek to discover some *change* in the pupil's established pattern of movement, singling it out as a *new element* of movement or of neuro-motor organization in the pupil. The pupil will allow this to happen only if it is discovered *in a playful, exploratory way* and considered to be safe and without risk. It should not be dramatically different from the established pattern of action, and it should not startle or shock the pupil. Pain caused by any manipulation (or even associated with it) can only destroy the learning situation, producing defensive reactions (not necessarily conscious) that will counteract any readiness to explore new ways of action.

3. I would call a "new" element any of the following: *(a)* the pupil becoming aware that some tense muscle can be released, thus allowing new movements; *(b)* the pupil gaining a sensory insight (kinesthetic or other) concerning behavior patterns; *(c)* the pupil finding a way to increase tonus in a muscle or in a muscle group that, for whatever reason, could not formerly be used or differentiated.

4. A new element in the above sense might emerge from a habitual pattern (a pattern of movement formerly allowed by the pupil), the element being "innocently" *added* to the pattern being changed. A nondifferentiated movement such as this, by associating and combining the new element of movement with a habitual one, avoids any suspicion or mistrust on the part of the pupil's nervous system. After a few repetitions of the movement one can assume that the added element, or rather the pupil's representation of it, has established itself as

possible and feasible. Now the new element can be singled out by a differentiated movement and further clarified by gently separating and distinguishing it from the other pattern.

5. I should mention that a limited range of movement patterns are often brought about by actual self-constraints (avoidance patterns or "anti-patterns") of which the person is mostly unaware. One might find, for example, tense muscles being "on the alert," or ready to interfere with the least hint of movement. We obviously cannot lead the pupil in a direction that goes against such a constraint. The new element will rather be found by exploring a movement that is not being resisted, perhaps a movement at right angles to the one being avoided, or it might be discovered in some "new combination" of elements. The image of that combined movement may be perceived by the pupil as "something unusual," but since it is being done gently, it should succeed in arousing the pupil's curiosity, which will obviously create a good learning situation.

6. Suppose now that a "new element" has been made clear within a definite context, fitting into a definite situation or serving some definite purpose. If it is left as an isolated, sporadically perceived experience, then it might be easily forgotten. It would hardly stand a chance of being assimilated into the pupil's normal ways of functioning. The pupil should be given the opportunity to familiarize himself with this new element, to make it something obvious and well understood. This means, of course, that we have to lead the pupil through different movement patterns, clarifying through these *different contexts* the role of this new element. These different contexts or *variations* will ultimately succeed in establishing a change in the pupil's "image of achievement." Success will be achieved more readily if we can show the relevance of that element to functions that are felt to be important and biologically vital.

7. Introducing a new element may also involve changing the initial position of the pupil's body. The teacher will decide whether to exhaust all possibilities latent in the initial position or to change over to an alternate one. For the sake of variation

in context, one might produce the same movement in a different orientation, for example, changing the pupil from lying on one side to lying on the back. Such changes in body position constitute a different pattern of movement or of action, because the muscular pattern will change with this change in spatial orientation. The environment and the direction of gravity, as perceived through the respective sensory channels, are components of any ongoing pattern of action; thus, with a simple change in orientation, there is already a change in the inner representation of that action.

8. Sometimes the teacher may decide to digress from the main procedure in order to clarify a detail or some other element encountered during the establishment of the new element's role. After having worked on that "side branch," the teacher shifts the interest again to the main "trunk." Occasionally, the teacher might decide to change the emphasis and postpone dealing with the first new element, following up to the end the functions of a second newly discovered element.

9. As in any effective learning, there comes a point at which it is useful to *sum up*, to review what has been learned. Summarization enables the pupil to recognize the new experience, the new insight, or the new knowledge all at one time, to feel it as something clear and simple. A concise *reminder* of the change expected to be assimilated is thus presented to the pupil. Any easy, playful movement, quickly and efficiently performed, that results from the foregoing, may serve this purpose. Sometimes a slight, well-placed support or pressure by the teacher's hands enhances the function of the new element by producing changes in the relative orientation of the body parts. This will have a summing-up effect. It is called the "clé de voûte" (or the keystone) in Feldenkrais parlance, because it is the central building block holding the newly learned pattern together.

10. It is clear that the teacher should not approach a lesson as if it were a tour that has been programmed in advance, with all the trails and roads chosen and with a definite goal in mind.

It should rather be an *exploring tour,* during which the goals might change at any time, according to the findings and to the pupil's responses.

11. Experience shows that if a session is done efficiently, without irrelevant manipulations and unnecessary digressions, it should not last more than thirty-five to forty-five minutes. The amount of really new information that the pupil's system is apt to assimilate at one time is limited, and after some time the teacher will notice that the pupil is not "there" anymore; a kind of fatigue occurs, although it is not physical in nature. We might suppose that the parts of the brain concerned with the programming of intentional actions have worked n ore than usual. It is preferable therefore to avoid any fatigue th it might otherwise cut short the effect of the summing-up pr)cess.

12. A tentative *plan for the next lesson* is like y to evolve in the teacher's mind during the latter part of th lesson. One might start by checking to what extent the new el ement is now less "new" and more integrated in the pupil's nor nal functioning. Sometimes the pupil may report verbally abo ut what happened between sessions, such as having moved d fferently, or having noticed changes in posture or self-image The lesson can then proceed with more variations (in the sen e of par. 6), starting perhaps with a new position and followe d by "sidebranches."

Let us now sum up what has been said about the structure of a lesson in Functional Integration:

While exploring and checking basic patterns characteristic of the pupil, the teacher *introduces a new element* that has hitherto been unclear, avoided, or nonexistent in the pupil's image of achievement, but which, nonetheless, is essential for reprogramming his neuro-motor patterns.

The teacher leads the pupil into experiencing *various contexts* in which the new element is relevant (such as diverse patterns of movement) and in which the element enhances efficiency, change, and vitality. At this stage, digressions may be made in order to clarify other new elements that may have been discovered along the way.

Summing up in a succinct way the role of the new element by initiating an easy, agreeable movement will enhance and clarify the various patterns that teacher and pupil have gone through, serving as a pleasurable reminder of the change.

The next chapter will present a few ideally conceived lessons that will help illustrate the content of the present chapter in a more tangible manner. These can serve also as schematic model lessons, to be eventually used in practice.

9. Schematic Outlines of a Few Model Sessions

The schematic descriptions outlined here are not intended to be followed and repeated as exact formulas. They should serve merely as starting points and then be adjusted to the special needs of the pupil. The various *initial positions* are chosen in order to satisfy, first of all, the pupil's requirement for comfort and safety, and secondly, the teacher's ability easily to produce movements affecting particular neuro-motor functions. What is said here about initial positions should not be taken as invariable procedure. Fully mastered, the technique is supposed to be carried out and developed so as to enable the teacher to work from any possible position.

The *order* in which the manipulons appear in these descriptions has a definite logic, but in actual practice there will always be differences in emphasis and in the choice of manipulons. If there is, for example, a problem in some distal part, then it is advisable to start with manipulons dealing with the corresponding proximal part, and vice-versa. Sometimes only a part of one of these sessions is carried out, and sometimes the sequence is interrupted in order to proceed with something else, according to the determinations of the teacher.

Exploratory manipulons, although essential, will receive little mention here, for the simple reason that they vary in each case. If the teacher chooses to carry out only a part of one of these sessions, there should nevertheless be a summing up with appropriate integrating manipulons, in accordance with what has been said in the previous chapter.

It is not necessary to define precisely the quantitative parameters of manipulons, such as velocity of movement, amount of force used, extent and precise direction of movement, or number of times a movement is repeated. With increased experience the teacher will refine the ability to determine these factors.

The fact that the following descriptions will deal more with movement (the active part of the manipulons) is not to be taken as an indication that the active part is more important than other factors we have mentioned. The exploratory and playful character of the manipulons in general, and the emphasis on bi-directional communication are both predominant features of the method.

The sessions described here are not intended to be carried out one by one in the order in which they appear. This order has no special significance; the numbering of the sessions is merely for the purpose of identifying them for future reference.

Session 1: Clarifying the Connection of Pelvis and Thorax (side position)

The pupil lies on one side. In order to be specific, we will assume it is the left side. An appropriate, soft support underneath the left ear will allow the neck to be aligned comfortably with the spinal column. The knees, bent approximately at a right angle, are lying one on the other. The thighs are bent at the hip joints, approximately at a right angle as well. The arms are placed one on the other so that the hands are somewhere in front of the face. This position is similar to the fetal position.

A slight push on the right-side process of the seventh cervical vertebra in the direction of the pelvis, applied simultaneously with a helping push (if needed) on the top of the head, allows one to check the functional connection between the pelvis and the rest of the body. The same connection is checked by the opposite movement—by pulling the head (fig. 13). This pull should be made in line with the cervical vertebrae. In more precise terms, the direction of the pull should coincide with the direction of the tangent of the cervical curve at its highest point (at right angles to the facets of the vertebrae), to avoid producing a shearing stress. No correction of either the placement of the head or its position in terms of flexion-extension is intended.

Now begin a clarification of the pelvis-thorax connection through the more distal parts that might possibly be involved. The shoulder and the shoulderblade are moved in the various cardinal directions: toward the pelvis and away, toward the vertebral column and away ("forward"), and over the underlying ribs in a kind of rotational (counter-clockwise) movement (the direction it would move, for example, when lifting the elbow "forward" and "up"). If necessary, emphasis can be put on the movement of the lower tip of the shoulderblade.

Next, the teacher holds the pupil's right arm horizontal to the

Fig. 13

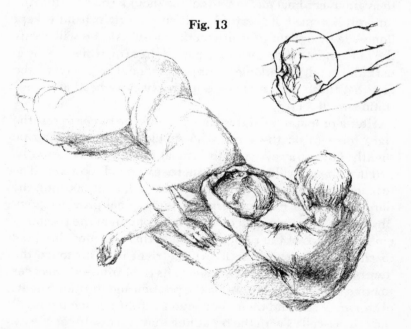

body by the elbow and lifts the arm up diagonally ("up" in the pupil's frame of reference), while touching with the other hand the pupil's right shoulderblade. The teacher can then shift that hand over from the shoulderblade to the vertebral column in order to emphasize its participation as well in this reaching-out of the right arm.

If the pupil has difficulty allowing the shoulderblade's participation in the arm's movement, this can perhaps be clarified by a relative conjugate movement in the following way: The pupil's forearm is propped up vertically on the table, so that the hand is at the level of the pupil's face. (If the required hyperextension of the wrist is difficult, then one can place only the thumb on the table, while the fingers go around the table's edge.) The teacher places his left hand on the pupil's elbow and his right hand on the shoulder just above the shoulder joint. Movements of the humerus along its own axis (at a right angle to the chest) can now be made and subsequently combined with the various cardinal movements of the shoulderblade, while the forearm is kept in its vertical position. The right hand is kept immobile by a slight pressure on the elbow. All this will clarify the movements of the proximal part of the arm, while the distal part (the hand) is motionless. Emphasis should be placed on the fact that these movements are made with the head and neck stationary (fig. 14).

After a preparation of this kind, it should be easier to rest the right forearm on the table. The shoulderblade will then be slightly farther away from the spinal column than formerly, and the head will assume a more extended position. The teacher now sits facing the pupil's back and, by supporting the dorsal vertebrae from underneath their spinal processes, emphasizes the participation of the spinal column in the reaching-out movement of the right arm. When this becomes clear, the teacher can then use the flat of the right hand to touch the lower border of the thoracic cage on its right front side in order to bring to the pupil's attention the position and the movements of the small ribs and their connection with the reaching-out of the arm as well as with the breathing movements. In the mean-

Fig. 14

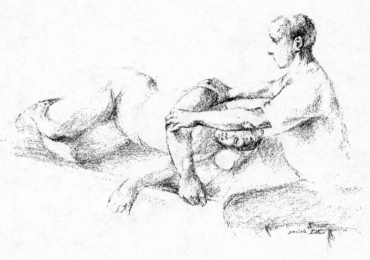

while, the vertebrae are supported from underneath, as outlined before, with the left hand (integrating manipulon).

Another integrating manipulon may be produced by extending the arm with the right hand in the manner outlined before,
while the left hand touches the greater trochanter (fig. 15). It is
possible in this way to pull the arm and push the pelvis in the
opposite direction alternately, or to produce these movements
simultaneously.

Still another integrating manipulon may be produced by
leaving the right arm on the table with the upper part of the
body in the slightly twisted position arrived at before, and placing the upper knee—the right one in this case—behind the
lower one. This is easily done by lifting the slightly extended leg
a little bit and alternately pushing and pulling the pelvis into a
rocking movement, "up" and "down." When this movement
can be made more or less easily, the right knee will descend to
the table easily and position itself behind the left knee. By
putting one hand on the shoulder joint and the other on the hip
joint, the teacher helps the pupil to become aware of the increased distance between these two joints and the ease with

Fig. 15

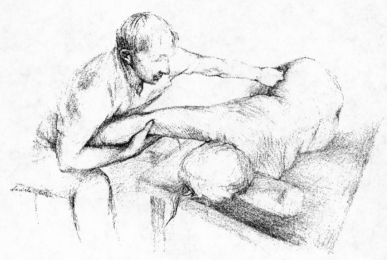

which the position is attained. It is even possible to draw the
pupil's attention to this situation verbally while juxtaposing it
with the habitual shorter distance between these two points.

In order to enhance this pattern a little more, the teacher can
do the following: Facing the pupil, the teacher places the part
of the right forearm near the elbow on the pupil's shoulder
joint and the left one on the hip joint, while the fingers of both
hands support the spinal processes from underneath. With
small movements the two joints are gradually pushed apart,
while the vertebral column is lifted with the fingers (fig. 16).

After this clarification of the twist forward of the upper part
of the body, together with the elongation of the right side of the
body, comes the opposite pattern: The right knee is returned
to its previous position, that is, aligned with the left one, or, if
this is feasible, the right knee is placed in front of the left one,
which is then shifted backwards slightly. The lower right leg
thus lies completely on the table. Putting the palm of one hand
on the pupil's forehead and taking the pupil's right elbow with
the other, the teacher turns the head with the arm and shoulder

Fig. 16

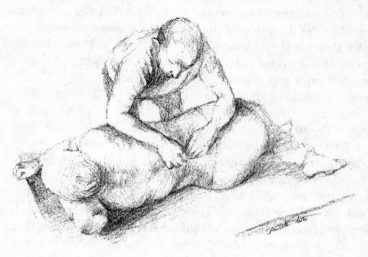

as one unit, as if to look up at the ceiling (a positioning manipulon, produced by a nondifferentiated movement). If this is not easily done, then a smaller change in position will suffice, and if the right knee was formerly on the table, it can be replaced on the other knee, so that the twist of the trunk will be less pronounced. There may be a need to pull the left arm, which is on the table, outward to the left, so that the left shoulderblade finds its place in this new position more easily.

A comfortable pulling of the right arm overhead (over the pupil's head), repeated a few times gently and without completely extending the elbow, may clarify the participation of the chest movement and the rocking of the pelvis in the reaching-out movement of the arm, but in a different direction than before. If the right shoulderblade does not participate easily in the movement of the arm described above, one can then either illuminate the situation by pushing the outer ridge of the scapula towards the spinal column, with the movement of the humerus down, or work with a smaller extension of the arm. After clarification the right arm can be pulled again.

Next, the teacher puts the pupil's right arm on the table

behind the back, with the knees remaining in the same position and the palm of the hand facing down (fig. 17). A slight push of the head in the direction of the cervical vertebrae, a direction actually slanting down toward the table, will further increase the twist of the upper part of the body to the right. The head is then left on a soft support, if this be needed.

Since the abdominal muscles, especially on the right side, may tense up because of the twist of the trunk, or perhaps they will have already tensed, one can ease this by substituting for the effort that they are making. This can be done by gently supporting the seventh cervical vertebra from underneath. Such a support can be nicely effective if the teacher holds with the left hand the pupil's head in a slightly flexed position, while supporting with the fingers of the right hand the seventh cervical vertebra from under the left side of its spinal process, so that a very slight lift is possible. This lift should be just enough to bring the small ribs on the right side slightly nearer to the pelvis (confining manipulon). A deep inhalation by the pupil will indicate that the tonus of the abdominal muscles has indeed diminished.

Fig. 17

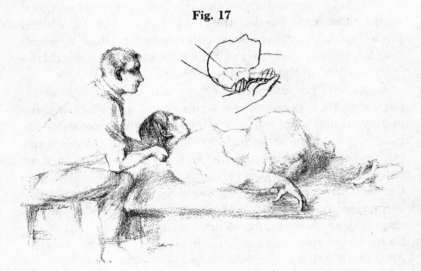

In this situation an integrating manipulon could be executed in the following manner: The teacher pushes the seventh cervical vertebra by its right-side process toward the pelvis, while taking with the left palm the pupil's jaw gently from underneath, as if hyper-extending the head, and both these movements alternate with each other in a rhythmical way, the right hand pushing towards the pelvis, the left hand pulling away from it. If these alternating movements can be changed into an oscillatory movement, then the pelvis should begin rocking with these oscillations. When this happens, the teacher can put the right hand on the pelvis and push it away, alternating the movement with the pulling of the jaw, as before. For the pupil this will produce the sensation that the entire vertebral column is moving in a chain-like manner. If this happens, it is worth drawing the pupil's attention to it verbally.

This new movability in the pelvis is so important that one should take further steps in integrating it. Facing the back of the pupil, who remains in this twisted position, the teacher puts the left hand, or the fingers of the left hand, underneath the spinal processes of the lower dorsal vertebrae, the right hand on the pelvis from above. By bringing these two places slightly nearer to each other, a substitution is made for the effort of the above-mentioned right-side abdominal muscles (confining manipulon). Usually there will be a deep breathing-in by the pupil.

The right arm can now be brought back to its initial position, as well as the right knee. The teacher places the hands, from above, one on the right side of the rib cage, one on the right side of the pelvis. Simultaneous pressure forward on the pelvis and backwards on the chest, which produces a twist in one direction, alternates with the reverse of these movements. Gently done, one can produce a slow oscillatory movement (watch the frequency!). This manipulon sums up the easy movability of the pelvis relative to the chest, or the equivalent movability of the chest relative to the pelvis.

As a final integrating manipulon, one can revert to the first manipulon done (p. 128), checking the movability of the pelvis by pushing the seventh cervical vertebra toward the pelvis or by pulling the head. The ease of the movement will be noticed, not only by the teacher, but also, one hopes, by the pupil.

As for the continuation of the session, there are two possibilities. The first is to repeat the same sequence on the other side. This should take place more easily and quickly, since the pupil will have already experienced the changes involved and can anticipate what is going to happen.

The other possibility is not to do the same on the other side, thus leaving the pupil with a sense of asymmetry. If this asymmetry is quite pronounced and obvious, then it may happen that the pupil will equalize both sides by himself, and this juxtaposition of both situations is an important experience in the pupil's learning process. Since the interest and the curiosity of the pupil are involved in comparing and discerning differences, the changes are being monitored and implemented through upper-level control. The experience of working this out for oneself, of discovering that one has the ability to transfer knowledge, is important in boosting the pupil's confidence in the ability to learn and to improve.

Session 2: Clarifying the Connection of Pelvis and Thorax (prone position)

The pupil lies on the stomach with the legs straight, the face turned to the left, and the left arm flexed comfortably, so that the hand is lying somewhere in front of the face. The right arm lies alongside the body. If there seems to be any difficulty in extending the ankles, a soft, round, foam-rubber pad should be put underneath them. The teacher explores the extensors of the back in order to find out what their tonus is. The feasibility of lifting up the left side of the pelvis is also explored. This lifting of the left side of the pelvis should render any sensation in the neck easier, twisted as it is, since it is partly undoing this twist. The slight rotation of the pelvis will become more evident if it is prepared by moving the distal part (the pupil's left leg). The teacher supports the left leg from underneath the ankle with the right hand and lifts it off the table so that the knee is bent at a right angle and the thigh is still on the table. Moving the lower leg back and forth ("left" and "right" in the pupil's frame of reference), the teacher brings the thigh into a rotating movement, to and fro, rolling around itself on the table—the range of this movement can be easily checked. The left knee is then shifted a very small distance toward the outside (a slight abduction of the thigh) and, while supporting the underside of the hip joint with the left hand, the teacher brings the leg down, so that it lies crossed over the pupil's right ankle.

This position can be established comfortably by slightly shortening the extensors of the back on the pupil's right side. This can be done by putting one palm on the ribs of the right side of the chest and the other on the right side of the pelvis, while standing in back of the pupil, and bringing them slightly nearer to each other.

It should be pointed out that in this movement, the right-side extensors of the back have as antagonists the left-side abdominal flexors. This is, by the way, an instance of *diagonal antagonism* between groups of muscles, which also occurs, in an analogous way, in movements of the head relative to the chest. The significance of this may become clearer to the pupil if the teacher simultaneously touches with one hand, from underneath, the edge of the rib cage near the abdomen on its left side, and with the other the anterior superior spine of the pelvis, which in this position is now lifted away from the table. This simultaneous touching of both the insertion and the origin of the left-side flexors of the trunk may clarify the greater distance between these two points, as well as the movement that occurs there during breathing (conforming manipulon).

An additional integrating manipulon may be produced by a slight pulling of the right hand downwards, combined with an easy outward rotation of the arm. This may be accomplished by placing the pupil's palm on the right buttock with a reaching-out movement, or pushing the seventh cervical vertebra through its right-side process in the direction of the pelvis, thus shortening the right-side extensors once more.

The latter movement may also be produced by simultaneously supporting the left shoulder with the right hand and touching—if it is feasible—the pupil's chin from below with the fingertips of the same hand, as if producing a slight extension of the head (fig. 18). This combined movement can be done either in a repetitive way or as a confining manipulon, which will ultimately evoke the reaction of a deep inspiration (especially pronounced on the pupil's left side).

After preparations of this kind, the pupil's left knee can be drawn up easily. The new element that facilitates this is the twist of the pelvis, which is equivalent to taking the hip joint "back" and "away." The teacher demonstrates this by supporting the hip joint with one hand and sliding the knee and the leg forward, so that the thigh is now flexed in the hip joint at approximately a right angle.

With this change in position, it is advisable now to check the neutral position of the head in terms of its forward-backward

Fig. 18

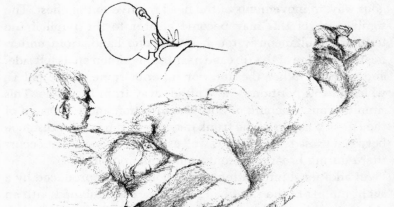

orientation as well as the flexing-extending balance. The teacher does this by placing the left hand around the base of the skull (on the back of the pupil's head) and the right hand around the base of the chin, so that the fingers will be nearer to the table from below, and the thumbs will touch from above. Arriving at the neutral position, the teacher can gently pull the head in order to check if such a pull is transmitted to the pelvis, or perhaps even to the right heel. This should be done with the utmost caution along the line of the cervical vertebrae, and the chin is not to be lifted, in order to avoid increasing the twist of the cervical spine.

The left leg is now extended again and the right arm is brought forward symmetrically with the left one. The turning of the head is now prepared by slightly lifting both shoulders from underneath, alternately as well as simultaneously, while noticing the sliding of the scapula over the rib cage. This can serve as a juxtaposing manipulon, since the pupil has the opportunity to compare the forces by which both shoulders are being sustained and, perhaps, to relax the extra effort in the right shoulder, similarly to that in the left one. Now the head is turned to the other side with the utmost care, with the teacher holding and slightly pulling it. Barely lifting the head up from the table with the fingers will enable the teacher to tuck in, so to speak, the pupil's chin (held by the right hand underneath the throat), so that the head is now straight and the neck untwisted (beware of hyper-extending the neck or of touching the throat). From here onwards the turn can be completed, either with the hands in the same position on the pupil's head, or by interchanging the positions of the hands.

After this complex positioning manipulon comes a simpler one, which is performed by placing the left arm alongside the body. Sometimes the turning of the head presents no problem at all and, if this is the case, the pupil can simply be asked to turn the head to the other side unaided.

The teacher continues by repeating the same sequence on the other side.

Session 3: Clarifying the Connection of Pelvis and Thorax (supine position)

The pupil lies on the back with both arms alongside the body, the knees drawn up so that the feet are planted on the table at a reasonable distance one from the other, approximately shoulder-wide. Sitting at the pupil's head, the teacher places his fingers underneath the shoulderblades and checks the ease with which these can be lifted up from the table. He also checks the possibility of pushing the seventh cervical vertebra slightly upwards, or to the sides, or diagonally from each side in the direction of the opposite knee. It is not meant that the seventh cervical vertebra should move relative to the neighboring vertebrae, but rather that the entire region of the vertebral column should yield slightly and elastically to such pressure.

The possibility of moving the pelvis and the lumbar spine can be checked in an analogous way. The teacher sits facing the pupil's right hip joint and pushes the right greater trochanter from underneath, towards the right shoulder (fig. 19). While doing this with the right hand, he pushes the right anterior crest of the ilium with the left hand, slanting it diagonally across the front of the body as if bringing it nearer to the left shoulder. He repeats this checking of pelvic and lumbar movements on the pupil's left side.

Improvement in the quality of these proximal movements will also be checked during this session by observing appropriate movements of the distal parts of the body.

The teacher extends the pupil's legs and places the feet slightly apart in a comfortable manner. Standing near the pupil's left hip joint, he takes the pupil's right arm and pulls it gently in a diagonal direction, as if toward a point situated vertically above the left hip joint. This movement of the arm, if made in the appropriate direction, should engage the shoulderblade. If the stretching out of the elbow is felt to be awkward, the teacher should take the arm in two places, at the forearm near the wrist and on the upper arm near the elbow, thus preventing the full extension of the elbow during the

Fig. 19

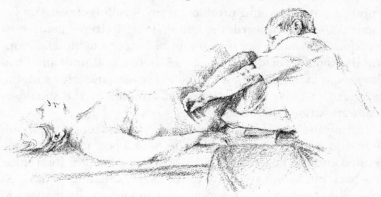

movement. If the pupil's shoulderblade doesn't seem to move easily enough, then the pull of the arm should be smaller, easier, and in a direction closer to the vertical.

Since the chest is somewhat involved in this movement of the arm, the necessity of differentiating this movement from the movement of the pelvis may arise. The teacher continues to extend the pupil's right arm, with the right hand only, and places the left hand on the right side of the pupil's pelvis in order to emphasize its immobility.

A similar situation may arise relative to the head. The pupil's head will roll with every pull of the arm in the same direction (to the left) in a nondifferentiated movement. The teacher can continue pulling the arm with the left hand only, while touching the left side of the pupil's head with the back of his right hand as a stop for the head's movement (confining manipulon). After a few movements done this way, the pupil may get the hint and become aware of the possibility of differentiating the movements of the shoulder from those of the neck.

The teacher sits again at the pupil's head, supporting the right shoulderblade from underneath. This should now be much easier to do than at the beginning. The pupil's right palm is placed on the pupil's left shoulder, so that the elbow comes to lie somewhere over the middle of the chest. Still supporting the right shoulderblade, the teacher puts his left hand on the pupil's right elbow and produces a small rolling-flexing movement of the chest towards the left hip joint. Extreme gentleness is required, because this movement may not be habitual. Grasping the shoulderblade by its "spine" between thumb and forefinger and fixing the elbow on the chest with the left hand, the teacher can make small sliding movements of the shoulderblade in various directions.

During all these movements, especially the lifting of the shoulderblade away from the table, the neck becomes slightly extended and the head hangs backwards. The teacher then shifts the back of the head slightly to the right, situating it "above" the right shoulder, a movement that induces a slight rotation of the head to the left (fig. 20). It is now possible, with each slide of the shoulderblade, to push the top of the head imperceptibly in the direction of the cervical spine, as if simultaneously arching and shortening the right side of the pupil's body.

The teacher still holds the right shoulderblade with the right hand in an elevated position and brings the pupil's head into its habitual, straight position. Taking the pupil's right elbow with the left hand, the teacher attempts to extend the humerus slowly over the pupil's head. Obviously, all of the foregoing has been a way of substituting for the effort of the right pectoral muscles and has probably decreased their tonus, so the extension of the right arm should be performed easily.

There is no need to obtain the full extension of the arm in a direct manner. It can be done through a relative conjugate movement in the following way: The teacher's left hand holds the elbow fixed in space at a place where the extension is easily reached, while the right hand shifts the shoulderblade toward the outside and up from the table, so that the shoulder joint becomes more extended with every repetition of this movement. Then the teacher can place the entire arm and the shoulderblade down on the table, the arm above the pupil's head, probably surprising the pupil by the ease with which this extension has occurred.

Fig. 20

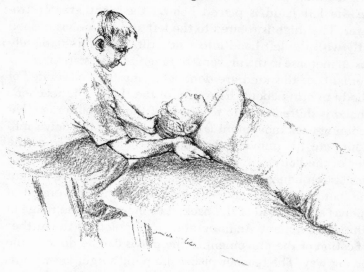

A few pulls of the straight arm will definitively establish the whole range of the extension, as well as the participation of the shoulderblade and the chest in the reaching-out movement of the arm.

The right arm is put back in its place alongside the body, and the same sequence is now repeated on the left side.

What has been accomplished relative to the chest through arm and shoulder movements can now be done with the pelvis, utilizing leg movements. Again, the knees are bent and the feet in the same position as at the beginning of the session. The teacher stands facing the right knee and lifts up the foot, so that the lower leg is horizontal and the thigh vertical. Holding the leg with both hands, the teacher checks the movements of the thigh in the cardinal directions, namely, in and out (adduction and abduction), up and down (flexion and extension), and rotation around itself.

To check the participation of the pelvis in this last movement, the teacher now holds the right leg with the right hand in a secure manner, perhaps by holding it close to his own body, while the left hand is placed behind the right greater trochanter. The thigh is rotated to the left and the pelvis pushed slightly with the left hand into a side tilt. This is immediately felt as an increase in the movement range of this rotation. A few movements of this kind are done, allowing the "elasticity" of the body to bring about the return of the thigh. The teacher's left hand is shifted over to the front of the trochanter, so that the coming-back movement is aided by pushing the pelvis into the opposite tilt (moving the right hip joint away from the center of the body).

This last sequence begins with what seems to be a movement of the foot to the left and right and ends with a movement of the pelvis at the small of the back, thus increasing the range of the initial movement. An integrating manipulon for the further clarification of the movement of the pelvis can be done in the following way: The teacher places the pupil's right leg with its slightly lifted knee against the planted left leg and, while leaving the right palm on the pupil's right knee, puts the right elbow over and around the pupil's left knee. In this way, the forearm can be used as a lever to turn the pupil's pelvis in a similar movement as before, but this time with the pupil's left leg serving as an axis. The teacher's left hand can push behind the pupil's right greater trochanter, in order to help in this movement (fig. 21). To do this in a comfortable way, the teacher might, for example, sit on the table, somewhere below the pupil's pelvis.

With the pupil still lying on the back, the teacher stands by the feet, the right hand on the pupil's right knee. Reaching out with the left hand for the pupil's left hand, the teacher orients it toward the right knee. The knee is now pushed diagonally towards the left shoulder, and this alternates with the pulling of the left arm towards the right knee. The alternating movement then changes into a simultaneous one, so that the pupil's trunk is *flexed and twisted* at the same time. After a few of these movements, the pupil can be shown how far he can reach out, with the teacher's help of course, with his left hand towards the right buttock, outside of the right thigh.

The above sequence is now carried out for the left side, using the other leg and arriving ultimately at the opposite twist of the trunk.

Finally, the teacher and the pupil will notice the ease by which both legs can be extended straight on the table. The analogy of what happened before with the extension of the arms should be also noted. Gentle pushes and pullings through each of the feet in the direction of the head, followed by checking the neutral position of the head with due attention to the breathing, conclude this session.

Session 4: Clarifying the Connection of Ankle and Knee Joints and Pelvis (supine position)

With the pupil lying on the back, the knees bent and the feet planted comfortably apart on the table, the teacher checks the functions of the ankle, observing first the alignment between

Fig. 21

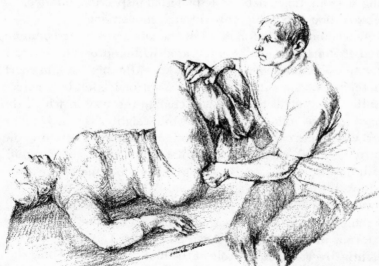

the leg, the ankle joint, and the foot, and any possible differences between left and right. The teacher now places a hand on one of the pupil's knees and grasps the malleoli between the thumb and finger of the other hand (the malleoli are the protruding round bones on each side of the ankle joint). Keeping the knee fixed in space, the teacher tries gently to move the ankle to the outside and back to the center, as well as to the inside and back, without sliding the foot on the table. In this way, the movability of the ankle relative to the *inversion* and *eversion* of the foot can be checked.

The teacher then extends the pupil's legs and holds one of them with one hand underneath the ankle in order to lift the heel slightly off the table. With the other hand, the movements of the foot at the ankle joint in the cardinal directions are now checked. This means flexion and extension as well as inversion and eversion. Sometimes it is advisable, instead of holding up the heel, to support it, as well as the knee, with some soft padding, in order to prevent hyper-extension.

Deviations from the efficient use of the bony structure of the leg are sometimes noticeable by visual inspection, but decisive observation is possible only through movement.

Deviations in the functions of the ankle are quite common, and any change must be integrated with appropriate changes in the use of the foot, the leg, the knee, the hip joint; in short, in the use of the entire body. Any disturbance felt by a person in the ankle or in the foot will change the way in which the person steps on the foot, transfers the weight of the body to the leg, walks, and carries out many other functions. Therefore, the help the pupil will get in reorganizing the ankle will be significant only if it is integrated with as many other motor functions as possible.

With the pupil still on the back, the teacher now turns the left leg slightly to the outside with the knee slightly bent, so that the external malleolus comes near the table. The ankle is thus slightly inverted and the sole of the foot can be seen. Some soft support underneath the knee from the outside may be necessary in order to diminish the strain on the adductor muscle. The teacher locates the navicular bone, which is slightly prominent in this position, located a little bit below and somewhat in front of the inner (medial) malleolus on the line joining the malleolus and the big toe. Gently pushing the navicular bone from below in the direction of the knee, but slanting the pressure slightly towards the table, will increase the inversion by making more use of the joint between the navicular and the talus. The talus bone is the uppermost bone of the foot; it articulates with the bones of the leg. At this point, one can gradually turn the foot with the other hand, grasping the base of the big toe.

The inversion of the foot usually comes with the outward rotation of the leg, and this element can be enhanced by adding, to the push on the navicular bone, a push of the head of the fibula toward the pelvis (fig. 22). The fibula is the more slender of the two bones of the leg, and is situated on the leg's outer side. The head of the fibula is situated immediately below the knee joint on the outside of the leg; it is easy to locate while the knee is slightly flexed, as it is here. This movement, a conforming manipulon, is made simultaneously, and although it is very small, it relieves some of the effort of the biceps femoris muscle —which is attached to the head of the fibula—and also defines clearly the direction in which the navicular bone can move. It should be pointed out that in this movement, the foot itself turns around its outer edge, which serves as an axis, fixed and supported by the table.

Having clarified this manipulon by a few repetitions, one can use the elastic coming-back movement in order to initiate the movement in the opposite direction. The big toe is then turned beyond the above-mentioned axis, as in turning the sole of the foot toward the table; the ankle shifts itself to the inside and the head of the fibula moves slightly away from the pelvis (eversion of the foot and inward rotation of the leg). While helping the head of the fibula to move away from the pelvis, one should proceed carefully, because of the possibility of pain. One should not press too hard on the foot either, and if this movement— however small—is not produced easily, it should be given up altogether. Whatever the result, the pulling of the head of the

Fig. 22

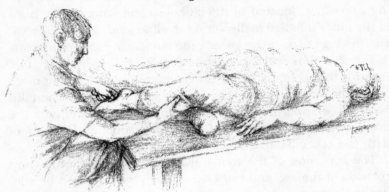

fibula away from the pelvis can at least be used as a way of pulling the pelvis itself into a diagonally rocking movement. Thus, one provides the pupil with a nonhabitual pattern of movement, involving the entire body and particularly the ankle.

Leaving the left leg as it is (slightly to the side), the teacher now takes the right leg, bent at the knee with the foot on the table, and tilts it to the inside, towards the other leg. Such a position will be possible only if the right hip joint works easily and the pelvis comes into a slightly extended and twisted position. In order to facilitate this for the pupil, one should do it only to the point where it does not call for any special effort, and at this point one pushes the pelvis back by pushing the knee along the line of the thigh towards the hip joint (confining manipulon). This provides a substitution for the effort of the muscles connecting the pelvis with the chest. An oscillatory movement of the pelvis, produced by pushing the knee in an appropriate manner, is also possible. This pressure can be applied through both knees at the same time. The right knee can then be lowered onto the table in this position. If this is still difficult, a soft support in between the legs should be provided.

The teacher now stands behind the pupil's head, takes the pupil's hands in his, extends the arms diagonally above the pupil's head, and pulls the right arm slightly so that the chest, the pelvis, and the knees come into a rocking movement (fig. 23). The left arm is then pulled in a similar way, while the teacher observes and compares what can be seen and felt on both sides. Differences are to be expected, mainly because of both knees being tilted to the left. Both arms can be pulled simultaneously as well. A slight pull of the head will produce a similar movement in the pelvis (integrating manipulons).

The arms are replaced alongside the body, the legs are straightened out, and the same sequence is repeated with the other leg and ankle.

Session 5: Clarifying the Connection of Ankle and Knee Joints and Pelvis (prone position)

The pupil lies on the stomach with the legs extended and the face turned to the side that seems more comfortable (in case there is such a preference at all). Let us assume that the face is turned to the left. The arms will assume a comfortable position, with the left arm bent forward, so that the left hand comes somewhere in front of the face, and the right arm straight back alongside the body. The teacher sits at the pupil's feet and lifts the left ankle with both hands, so that the knee, supported as it is by the table, is slightly bent. This position should allow easy movement of the ankle and heel to the left and right.

There are two possibilities in this position: one is to keep the leg in space while turning the *lower leg* around itself (rotating it around its own axis, which is usually a very restricted movement); the other possibility is to move the ankle left and right in such a way that the entire leg up to the hip joint will move as one piece. The teacher has to allow the heel to move in a certain arc, so that the *thigh* will roll around itself on the table. The only working joint in this second movement will thus be the hip joint. In the pupil's representation, these two patterns may not be very well differentiated, both being related to the same *distal heel* movement (left and right). It is possible, therefore, to make an easy transition from one of these two patterns to the other, either by turning the lower leg around itself and changing to the rotation of the entire leg and hip joint, or by

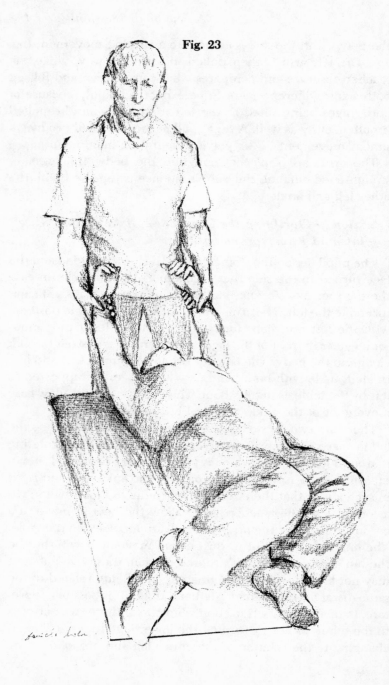

Fig. 23

executing the two movements in reversed order, whichever seems the easier.

When these movements become clarified, the teacher can shift the pupil's left knee slightly to the outside and, holding the foot raised, with the knee in a somewhat flexed position as before, can try rotating the thigh around itself again. It may turn out that, while rotating it to the inside, the heel comes nearer to the table than before. The teacher determines which angle of the knee joint allows the greatest lowering of the foot to the table, while turning the leg to the inside (to the right). When the big toe touches the table, the teacher uses it as a support for the foot and gently pushes the outside edge of the sole of the foot towards the pupil's head, slanting the movement down slightly, so that the heel comes nearer to the table and the hip joint lifts itself up (fig. 24). In this movement, the entire leg acts as a lever, with the fulcrum at the point where the knee touches the table. Notice that this movement has as a component a slight eversion of the foot. After a few repetitions, one does this movement as a confining manipulon, which usually obtains as a response a deep inhalation.

Fig. 24

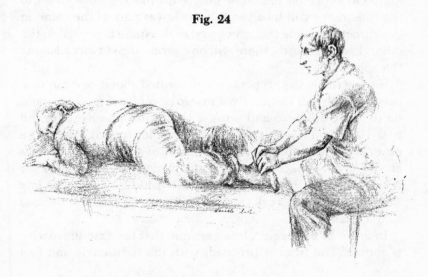

Eventually, the teacher moves the left knee a little bit more to the outside, and then proceeds with the left/right movement of the heel, lowers the foot to the inside and then tries again the lever-like movement, bringing the ankle down towards the table and the side of the pelvis up, and ending with a confining manipulon.

A few gradual steps of this kind will bring the knee up, flexed and to the side, with the hip joint away from the table and the chest, and the inside of the leg lying on the table.

It is important that the pelvis begin lifting in association with pressure through the sole of the foot, as part of a pattern akin to stepping on the leg or going up a stair, but isolated from other gravitational actions usually called for in an erect posture.

The leg can now be straightened out, the head and arms positioned on the other side, and the same sequence repeated with the other leg.

It should be pointed out, though, that in many instances it would be more helpful to continue this session in a different way, namely, to carry out the described sequence with the same leg, while the head, and correspondingly the arms, are positioned as above on the other side. With the knee drawn up to the side, there will be a twist in the lower part of the spine in one direction, while the upper part of the spine is twisted in the other. In other words, there will be a pronounced twist all along the spine.

Having made the preparations described above, one can proceed towards this further twist in two possible ways. One would be to leave the head and arms as they were (the head turned to the left), and then to work on the other leg (the right leg). The other possibility would be to turn the head and change the arms accordingly—especially since it might not be comfortable for the pupil to continue with the neck twisted for so long to one side—and again to work through the same leg (the left one), as in our example.

In order to be specific, let us assume that the first alternative is chosen. The teacher proceeds with the right ankle and foot this time, being more careful with the gradual shifting of the right knee to the right, because of the increased twist produced in the spine. When the right hip joint lifts itself off the table sufficiently, one puts the pupil's right arm, which is lying alongside the body, into the gap formed underneath the hip joint (fig. 25).

Having brought the knee to its final drawn-up position, the teacher explores the curvature of the spine. The line of the spinal processes of the vertebrae will now have two arcs, one with its convexity to the right (in the upper dorsal part) and one to the left (in the lumbar part). These should be located by the teacher and eased up from the concave side, so that the arcs become slightly increased, the upper arc more to the right, with its twist, the lower more to the left with its opposite twist. As an integrating manipulon, the teacher places the right palm underneath the pupil's left shoulder and clavicle, in position for lifting up the shoulder from the table, and the left palm underneath and behind the pupil's right thigh, near the pelvis, where the pupil's right hand is situated (fig. 26). He lifts both these

Fig. 25

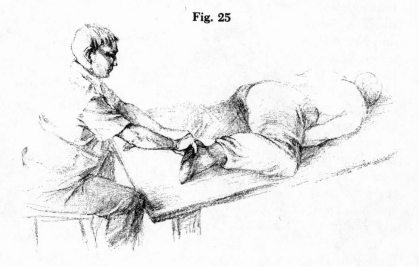

parts, alternately, and also at the same time, in a very gentle way. This will increase the already existing twist in the spine. The head should be also checked, by pushing it slightly in the direction of the cervical spine, as well as by pulling it. The appropriate direction for these movements must be chosen, or rather discovered, in a most gentle and careful way.

The right hand is now taken out from underneath the hip joint and placed forward, symmetrical with the left one. The head is turned to the right, and the left arm is turned back alongside the body. This positioning manipulon will be felt by the pupil to be a "coming home" towards a known and comfortable position.

The head is checked again as to its neutral position, and the right leg is straightened out.

Leaving the upper part of the body turned to the right, the teacher now carries out the appropriate sequence with the left leg, which leads finally to an increased twist in the opposite direction. The untwisting that follows, similar to the above pro-

Fig. 26

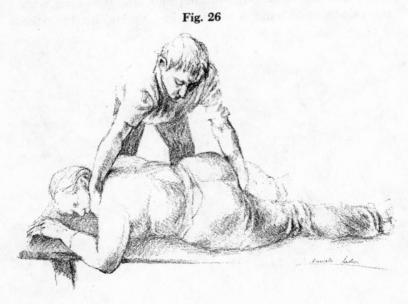

cedure, will leave the pupil's head turned this time to the left, as it was at the beginning of the session.

At the end of this session, the pupil's manner of sitting, as well as the manner of turning around to the left or to the right in order to look backwards (while sitting) should be checked; in other words, one checks to what extent the pupil is ready to utilize the twist in the trunk in everyday activities. One checks the way the pupil walks and to what extent he allows the pelvis to move.

Session 6: Clarifying the Connection of Pelvis and Thorax (kneeling position)

The pupil kneels on the floor, with the knees slightly parted in a comfortable way, next to the table and facing one of its sides. With the thighs upright, the stomach and chest are positioned across the table. A soft padding underneath the knees is necessary. The height of the table should be such as to allow the weight of the pelvis to be supported, at least partly, by the knees. The pupil's head is turned to the more comfortable side, and the arms are placed accordingly. For example, if the head is turned to the right, then the right arm will be flexed and the hand placed somewhere in front of the face, while the left arm lies alongside the body.

In this position, the pupil's pelvis can be easily moved in the cardinal directions, and its movability observed. The pelvis is, after all, the "most proximal" part of the body, at least in the prevailing kinesthetic representation. In this position all the movements of the pelvis will be relative conjugate movements, in respect to most of the habitual movement patterns of the pupil.

Characteristically, the hip joints are not extended, and, therefore, do not feel threatened, and the muscles in the small of the back are relieved of any necessity to engage in antigravitational patterns. The one aspect of the pupil's comfort that should be noticed particularly is the position of the neck. If the side rotation of the head is not comfortable for the pupil and the session is nevertheless considered important, both the pupil's hands can be put on the table with the forehead resting on them. The feet should be extended, and if this presents any difficulty, a soft roller can be placed as a support underneath the ankles.

The verticality of the thighs (as seen from the side) should be checked, so that the pupil will feel the pelvis to be safely supported by the thigh bones. In this way no sliding of the knees forward or backward will occur. If this is not the case, the knees should be shifted accordingly. The thighs, as seen by the teacher from behind, should be vertical as well, unless the table is too low (or the pupil too tall); in this case, the thighs are spread slightly. The weight of the pelvis should be distributed equally on both knees; otherwise, the pupil might be compelled to make a muscular effort (not on a conscious level) to hold the pelvis. A symmetrical stance of the thighs is necessary for this, and one can either shift the pelvis sideways, if that is feasible, or correct the position of one of the knees. Often these adjustments, by themselves, will enable the pupil to allow easy movements of the pelvis.

Next, the teacher sits behind the pupil, and studies the characteristic features of the pelvis's skeletal parts, since these will be used further to explore the movement patterns of the pelvis. The teacher finds the two greater trochanters from the sides, from behind, and from above, as well as the ischia (the sitting bones), which might be located in this posture at the level of the trochanters, but more to the inside. Exploration of the ischia shows that these are not just two pointed bones, but two flat and almost vertical bones with rounded edges. The distance between the two ischia is different in different persons, and will generally be larger in women. Then comes the exploration of the sacrum, with the line of the spinal processes of the sacral vertebrae and the two archlike ridges of the pelvic bone (posterior superior iliac crests) opening towards both sides.

All these explorations should be done in a very gentle way, as one may encounter quite a few painful spots.

Since the habitual patterns of the pelvic movements are

flexion and extension, and since any possible anti-patterns might therefore be directed against these, the patterns of flexion and extension should be explored last.

Let us suppose that the pupil's face is turned to the right. The right ischium can then be pushed from behind in a forward direction with a slight upward slant by the teacher's right hand, while the left hand helps simultaneously by pushing behind the left iliac crest towards the center of the trunk (fig. 27). The teacher leaves both hands in place and relinquishes the pressure. This will allow the "elasticity" of the system to produce the coming-back movement. The optimal direction for this diagonal movement of the pelvis, in terms of the pupil's comfort, will only be found with the utmost gentleness. After a few movements, the teacher can place the right hand above the right ischium, so that, by pushing the ischium down vertically, the coming-back movement is aided (fig. 28). A see-saw-like movement is now easily produced by alternating the pressure

Fig. 27

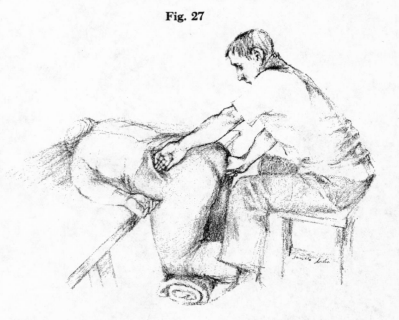

of the two hands. This movement has as an axis a line going through the hip joints. It might turn out that the downward movement of the ischium is not precisely vertical, but slightly slanted towards the middle.

A similar sequence is then carried out on the other diagonal, with the left ischium and the right iliac crest.

After elucidating both these diagonals, it is worth checking the straight-line movements, first the extension of the back, by pressing both ischia simultaneously in a forward direction with a slight upward slant, or by pushing both iliac crests from behind simultaneously, in a forward direction with a slight downward slant (confining manipulons). The opposite movement will be to press both ischia down vertically with the fists from above, which will produce a slight flexion of the pelvis and a lever-like movement, with the hip joints as pivots. In a different manner, the same flexion can be produced by gently supporting the

Fig. 28

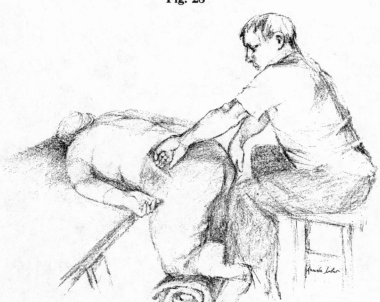

anterior iliac spine from underneath with the fingers of both hands, (confining manipulons). Obviously, such a slight flexion of the pelvis shortens the abdominal muscles, while relieving some of their effort, and lifts the lumbar spine slightly. The diaphragm becomes free and the response is usually a deep breathing-in that engages the small ribs of the back.

Next, the teacher faces the pupil's right side and checks the feasibility of increasing the spinal curve towards the left, in accordance with the already curved state of the upper spine, which has been produced by the position of the head. The increased flexibility of the spine will now become apparent. Increasing that curve is done by bringing the ribs and the pelvis nearer to each other on the right side, slightly pushing the vertebrae at different levels towards the pupil's left, and checking the easy movability of the shoulderblade and the shoulder in various directions (integrating manipulons).

The teacher then sits behind the pupil's head and deals with the integration of the head, neck, and shoulders with the changes produced in the organization of the spine. This includes checking the position of the head (forward and backward, extension and flexion), finding its neutral position, and applying slight pulls on the head in the direction of the cervical spine.

The head is now turned to the other side, and the position of the arms changed accordingly. The entire sequence is now repeated, with appropriate interchanges left and right. Attention should be paid to which of the two diagonal movements of the pelvis should come first.

The session may conclude at this point, or one can ask the pupil to lie on the back on the table, with knees bent and the feet planted on the table. Now one can add a few more integrating manipulons as desired (fig. 29).

One usually recognizes the functions one can deal with in the various initial positions as well as in schematically outlined sessions such as these. Ultimately, the teacher acquires the ability

Fig. 29

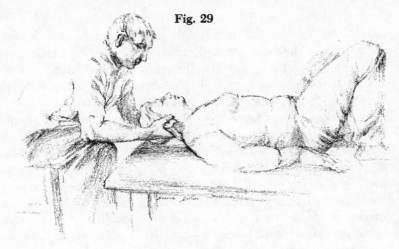

to choose the sessions or the various sequences of manipulons according to these specific functions. More often than not, however, this "decision" regarding which functions will be dealt with must evolve from an exploratory approach. Moreover, one's preconceived notions in this respect are bound to change, sometimes sharply.

Quite a few manipulons described in the foregoing chapters have not been part of the sequences described in the present chapter. The inventive teacher will devise still other schematic sequences, according to the already stated principles of a session's structure. It should be mentioned again that these sessions are supposed to be tried first on healthy people, members of the family or close friends, and that one should always keep in mind the gentle and nonintrusive character of Functional Integration.

10. A Few Typical and Often-Encountered Manifestations of Inefficient Neuro-Motor Organization

Suppose it were possible to have complete knowledge of the *functional nature* of a person's neuro-motor system—all of one's habitual and intentional patterns, as well as one's ways of adapting to various conditions, such as learning and creating. Were this possible we would have a fairly exact picture of the living character and individuality of this person. The variety of functional differences is as vast as the variety of human individuals; a functional richness so immense in scope we cannot grasp it.

If the nature of a particular person's neuro-motor system is in some way unsatisfactory, there is usually *something conspicuous* about it, something which might attract the teacher's attention, or of which the person might be especially aware.

This chapter deals with a few typical examples of inefficient neuro-motor organization, each defined by a prominent trait, and with the ways the teaching process might be started. When the teacher asks what would be the most helpful for the pupil, any specific detail relating to this pupil's functioning could be of utmost importance. In this respect, every person is a "category" unto himself. No two persons can be put in the same category, when we think of all that has happened in their lives, and of the diversity in their habits, expectations, and associations, all of which are functionally important.

On the other hand, let us compare two apparently disparate cases: a ten-year-old girl who has functional impairment in one of her hands, after having suffered from polio in her early childhood, and a fifty-five-year-old man with a functional disability in one of his hands, after having suffered a mild stroke. Typically, the disability in the distal part will bring about increased effort in the proximal parts (the muscles around the shoulder and upper arm will display a rigidity that is not due primarily to neurological changes in themselves). The teacher might propose similar things to both individuals in order to bring this extra effort towards upper-level control and thus to open the road for possible improvements in the ability to use the hand.

In any case, applying conclusions from one case to another when there is some similarity is not to be avoided; just the contrary. After all, this is one of the ways in which we learn by experience.

A warning should be made at this point: People classified in one or another of these categories should, in certain instances, be considered clinical or medical cases and the medical problem is not always related to the most prominent feature of inefficient functioning.

It should be said again very clearly that the approach of Functional Integration is absolutely nonmedical. If there seems to be the slightest indication of any medical problem, the person should of course be referred to a medical doctor. If a person is under current medical supervision, or is undergoing medical treatment—a fact that must be ascertained from the start— then there is no way of relating to him by this method, unless of course it is done in close collaboration with, and with the explicit consent of, the person's attending physician.

As has been said already, Functional Integration addresses only the way a person copes with structural or functional difficulties. The objective is not to diagnose, treat, and cure; it is, rather, purely educational.

The following are typical examples of inefficient neuro-motor patterns:

1. The Nonextending Trunk

A flexed trunk per se should not always be considered to be negative. If I have to lift something off the floor, one of the ways to do this is to bend my back. On the other hand, if I persist in being flexed as if intending to avoid stretching out or bending backwards, and if I am not even aware of the feasibility of extending my trunk, then I have a problem.

The first clue to such a state of affairs is provided by visual observation of the pupil's posture and movements. A more complete answer will be provided by exploratory manipulons to check the flexion and extension of the trunk. This checking of these functions might indicate that there are anti-patterns working against extension, that not only is one not using extension, but also that one is making an active effort to resist the possibility. In a case such as this, the flexors of the trunk are in a state of increased tonus most of the time.

The state of overworking flexors, concomitant with the inhibition of the extensors, was already mentioned in relation to the anxiety syndrome, but no premature conclusions concerning the causes of this state or the need to correct it should be drawn.

Clearly, no attempts at extension should be made against established anti-patterns. This would not clarify the situation for the pupil and would only increase the strength of the anti-pattern, which, after all, has become the habitual way of avoiding extension.

On the other hand, if we can create a situation in which the possibility of extension is sought *by the pupil* (so that the pattern is produced by the pupil's CNS in a different context from the one which elicits the anti-pattern), there may be a possibility for this pattern to be reinstated and accepted as an alternative to the stereotyped one.

The problem of the nonextending trunk may be addressed in

the following manner: with the pupil on one side, the teacher can start by substituting for the effort of the flexors of the trunk on one side only, clarifying low-level controlled functions related to these flexors (such as breathing, for example), as described in chapter 5.

One should take into consideration possible structural restraints, and not expect immediate, dramatic results. Sometimes it may seem that a dramatic change is occurring, but even then it may be transitory, since the pupil's CNS may not be ready to give up (at least on a nonconscious level) patterns of organization that may already have worked that way for a long time. Such patterns might be related to structural changes, as mentioned before, that have altered patterns of neuro-motor organization as a means of adapting to these changes. The CNS cannot be expected to simply revert to patterns of action appropriate to the "healthy" structure that was there *before* any changes occurred.

It is clear that any expected change will have to occur slowly and gradually. We do not expect a change in existing patterns, although this might occur subsequently. Progress will consist of clarifying alternatives to the existing patterns. The pupil's system will choose some of these alternatives only if they are felt to be comfortable and efficient; only then can one shed the compulsive and stereotyped way of acting.

After achieving some decrease in the flexors' tonus on both sides of the trunk, one can check the functions connected with the trunk's twisting as described in schematic session 1, or the diagonal movements (twist and flexion) in session 3.

The next stage might consist of working through the antagonists of the flexors (the extensors of the trunk) in one of the prone positions—lying on the stomach, or the kneeling position —and integrating the changes in the extensors with those in the flexors. Through this sequence some slight increase in lumbar lordosis (the forward curvature of the spine) might result as well as an improvement in the flexibility of the dorsal spine.

While the pupil is in a supine or sitting position, one can draw the pupil's attention to the movements of the small ribs on the front or on the sides as they occur during breathing. One could also lead the pupil to touch the rib cage with the flat of the hands in order to monitor its movements. It might then occur to the pupil that it would not be desirable to stop the ribs' movements. This insight is equivalent to diminishing the tonus of the abdominal muscles.

Rolling the pelvis forward while in the sitting position to produce an extension in the back and a slight lumbar lordosis might be very difficult for the pupil, since it is directly opposed to the prevailing anti-pattern that works against extension. On the other hand, asking the pupil to sit and look backwards over one shoulder might elicit the involvement of the small ribs on the other side more easily.

Still other patterns that do not involve extension directly could be proposed and tried out on both sides, until extension emerges as an obvious consequence of the foregoing.

This entire process, only briefly described here, is expected to be extended over a number of sessions so that the pupil can assimilate the clarifications and the corresponding sensory insights. The integration of this with other basic functions should be included in the learning process, namely, with the movements of the head, of the shoulders and shoulderblades, and of the hip joints. The movements of the pelvis as part of movement patterns of the extremities are important as well.

2. The Non-Twisting Trunk

I now propose an experiment to the reader that might clarify on a sensory level something which will be taken up later. Try to walk with very slow and small paces, while touching with the fingers of both hands the extensors of the back in the lumbar region, approximately at the height of the belt, on both sides of the spinal column. The palpating fingers will discover the alternating tensing up of the extensors, left and right, with every step. With each step, the corresponding extensor lifts the pelvis on the side on which the leg is lifted from the floor, and when the foot supports the weight of the body again the tension diminishes or subsides altogether.

This alternating activation of the extensors, on the left and on the right, is part of the pattern of walking, or more generally, of the pattern of shifting the weight of the body from one leg to the other. We are not usually aware of this pattern, since it is low-level controlled, being a pattern as old as our walking itself and thus an habitual pattern of the trunk. Considering that any muscular effort actually brings some muscle ends nearer to each other, one can see that having the weight of the body on the left foot, for example, and lifting the right foot off the ground, as in stepping forward, draws the right shoulder, or even the right side of the chest, backwards.

This is what actually happens in walking: when either of the legs makes its step forward, the ipsilateral shoulder goes backwards. This small alternating twist of the chest relative to the pelvis is quite familiar in a way, because everyone is aware of the swinging of the arms in walking, though it is low-level controlled, as was already noted.

The above-mentioned twist always occurs unless it is opposed and inhibited by some other pattern, which may quite often happen. Such inhibition by the abdominal muscles is in itself low-level controlled. In fact, pointing it out to a malfunctioning person might even not be helpful. One may not recognize the fact that a muscular effort that counteracts such a pattern is being made continuously. Often enough, this person might try to rationalize the situation by saying things such as "Am I really supposed to wiggle my body this way? Isn't that a little bit too sexy?" In other words, this person cannot envision permitting even the smallest movements in the trunk. The most minute twist is judged to be an exaggerated movement.

The *correction* that takes the pupil away from an extreme situation—whether it is actually done or only envisaged—is always *judged to be a deviation* towards the other extreme. The person's kinesthetic judgment, with all its related associations and connotations, is distorted by the habit and needs a recalibration, so to speak; a reassessment of what is feasible, acceptable, comfortable, and efficient.

The inhibition of the twist of the trunk will manifest itself not only in walking but in other functions as well. When attempting to clarify this situation, it is advisable to do it in relation to functions other than walking or standing, which might have their patterns too strongly established as integral parts of the person's self-image.

The abdominal muscles that are instrumental in producing this anti-twist pattern are working in a nondynamic way (tonic contraction); they are not producing movement or work. This inhibition is done only with a simultaneous activation of the extensors of the back (their antagonists) and therefore rigidity and lack of flexibility of the trunk is produced. This diminishes efficiency, interferes with good breathing (see chapter 5), and is tiring as well. Any movement produced occasionally by the trunk, such as bending forward to pick up an object, will thus be executed with constantly stressed and tired muscles that are contracted in spasm and pain and pressing the vertebrae towards each other. The trunk movements, if done at all, are produced without any twisting (with the trunk straight), which is not the most efficient way of using the trunk.

Various body training methods that put emphasis on strengthening the abdominal muscles might indeed bring about the strengthening of these muscles, but if one doesn't learn how to release them at the same time, the continuously stiff abdominal muscles become a restraining and bothersome element.

A *good* strong muscle is one that the person can use with any gradation ranging from the utmost power to complete relaxation. Such a muscle can have its force changed as the person wills, gradually or suddenly. Moreover, its differentiation from the activity of other muscles or any possible combinations of muscles should be easily perceived.

It seems that what we are expecting from a good muscle does

not reside in the muscle itself, but in the CNS, which directs the muscle to carry out various patterns of action, differentiated or complex as they may be.

Any clarification of the relationship between the pelvis and the thorax will be to the point and may be tried out. For example: The pupil lies on the back with extended legs, and the teacher pulls the pupil's right arm diagonally overhead. The pupil is asked to put the fingers of the left hand on the small ribs above the abdomen on the right side. In doing this, the pupil may become aware that, when the right arm is pulled upwards, these small ribs are moving up and away from the pelvis to some degree. The pupil is asked now to resist the teacher's pull without bending the elbow, all the while monitoring with the left hand the movements of the right-side ribs. This time the pupil will notice that the ribs are not moving up. When he stops the resistance, these ribs will again move up, perhaps even more than in the beginning. One can now draw the pupil's attention to the fact that when he pulls his arm down, the stomach muscles are mobilized in order to "anchor" the chest to the pelvis. The teacher may then ask whether the pupil considers this anchoring to be really necessary when he is not engaged in pulling down his arm. The insight may be striking and could help in bringing these patterns to the upper level of control.

Clarification of this nature should begin on the side on which movement seems easier, and then the juxtaposition of this side with the other one will be all the more impressive.

In order to show the pupil that this "anchoring" of the chest to the pelvis is to be used only for specific and limited actions, the teacher may ask that both heels be lifted one inch or so from the table (the legs still straight), so that this anchoring on both sides of the abdominal muscles (left and right at the same time) will become clear, this time as a muscular effort required for the intentional lifting of the legs. Breathing will stop while the legs are lifted and freed from the impeding action of the stomach muscles when the legs are lowered. If the teacher points this out, the pupil will be aware of the connection between the habitual rigidity and the breathing pattern, which predictably is not very satisfactory. These experiences may induce the pupil to attempt to consciously control the trunk muscles.

3. Scoliosis

The term "scoliosis" designates a sideways bend of the spinal column to one side. It is not meant to apply to any curvature that is produced intentionally, as this would constitute one of the normal ways of using the spinal column. The term applies to a permanent deviation, and one which is not under conscious control.

Much has been written about scoliosis, both as a medical problem and as a developmental one. The book on scoliosis by Cailliet* should be mentioned, as it makes the structural aspect of scoliosis especially clear. The book also surveys the current medical treatments for scoliosis.

Here we will deal with the neuro-motor aspect of scoliosis only, and with the way to achieve *improvement by increased self-awareness.*

The causes of scoliosis are generally not known, except in cases of congenital structural deformity or in neurological or neuro-muscular disorders, such as one-sided paresis and the like. In a great number of cases the scoliosis is discovered while the person is in his early teens, and worsens with time.

In the beginning the problem is an aesthetic one, but within a few years it can cause difficulties in movement, in breathing, and even in the functions of the inner organs.

From the start, there may be a factor which prevents the system from using the skeleton's antigravitational functions in the most efficient way—that is, from aligning itself properly for the various motor functions.

The question of alignment of the vertebrae is not a simple

* Rene Cailliet, M.D., *Scoliosis: Diagnosis and Management* (Philadelphia: F. A. Davis Co., 1975).

one. It is of course incorrect to think of the vertebrae merely as a row of small cubes stacked one over the other, which, when out of line, will simply collapse. The vertebral column is rather to be likened to an elastic, flexible stick which can be bent like a bow by a tense string.

Tense and shortened muscles can usually be found on the concave side of the arc-like part of the vertebral column forming the scoliosis. Whatever initially produced this muscular pattern is not particularly relevant once the scoliosis has developed, because the basic fact is that it has become a habit and is therefore low-level controlled.

The muscles that are instrumental in maintaining the deformation are not necessarily near the vertebral column. We have to consider, for example, that any pair of ribs articulated with the corresponding dorsal vertebra may act as a pair of levers on this vertebra and that muscles or any other forces acting on the distal parts of these ribs, because they possess great leverage, can directly change the orientation of this vertebra.

A few circumstances may further complicate the situation. The fact that the ribs are slanting downwards means that the muscles sustaining the deformation are not on the same level as the corresponding site on the vertebral column where the deviation is to be found. The latter is of course located higher than the former. For example, there might be a convexity to the left in the middle dorsal section of the spine somewhere in between the shoulderblades, while the muscles engaged in holding this deviation are the right-side abdominal muscles and the right quadratus lumborum muscle (see fig. 30).

Considering that the head, as the site where the teleceptors are located, should be held in a way that enables it to turn around a vertical axis, it is also possible that a compensatory curve may develop in the upper part of the vertebral column (the upper dorsal and the cervical spine) with its convexity to the right.

With the constant activation of the right abdominal muscles, the extensors of the left side in the small of the back are often

Fig. 30

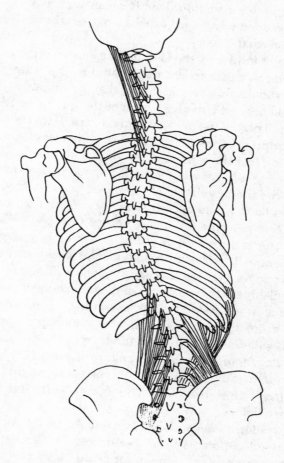

found to be tense as well ("diagonal antagonism" of this kind was mentioned in the previous chapter). Yet, here they are working together, not with reciprocal inhibition as efficiently functioning antagonists usually do.

The tense left-side extensors of the lumbar spine might be instrumental in maintaining the lumbar deviation with the convexity to the right, which might be considered a compensatory mechanism to the leftward dorsal deviation as well. Describing such a situation doesn't mean that it is easy to state what preceded what, what caused what, or what is the compensation for what.

Finally, considering the fact that the various muscles engaged in holding this pattern are not located in the same plane surface, it should not be surprising that a scoliosis of the kind described here will involve a twist of the spine, this twist being an integral part of the neuro-motor pattern. If we continue with the description of the schematic case which was begun earlier, we can see that the tension of the right abdominal muscles will draw the right lower ribs forward. This alone produces a slight twist of the thorax relative to the pelvis in a counter-clockwise direction (as it would appear when observed from above).

Now this person's self-image comes into play. Wanting to correct the picture as it is seen by looking at oneself in the mirror, one will draw the right shoulder backwards and push the left one forward, so that the line connecting the shoulder joints will appear to be parallel to the line connecting the hips.

If a process of this kind is started in the early teens while the growth process is still going on, what may happen is that the skeleton will develop with deviations from the normal, caused by the unchanging posture or even by pressure of the bones one on the other. For example, some vertebrae might assume a wedge-like shape, the two facets of the vertebral body not being parallel.

Such a deformity cannot be reversed. Any program of neuro-motor re-education will get better results the earlier it is started, or the nearer to the onset of the deviation.

The teacher may start by exploring the range of movement, ease of movement, and flexibility. Movements that are intended to "correct" the deviations should not be initiated; just the contrary. Movements that exaggerate the deviations can release the muscles engaged in maintaining the deviation, and when their tonus decreases, their contra-lateral antagonists, which have been inhibited most of the time, will now have a chance of increasing their tonus.

An example of this would be schematic session 5, which in its first part produces a scoliosis-like position.

Sometimes it seems easy to straighten the vertebral column of a young person with scoliosis while the person is lying horizontally. But this doesn't mean that this alignment will be preserved in a standing or even sitting position. The way that the system uses the skeleton in its antigravitational functions is in a certain sense faulty, as we discussed previously. The pupil's system does not align the vertebrae so as to make possible the propagation of forces through the skeleton without muscular effort, so the pupil should be provided with the experience of such a possibility. This can be done in almost any lying position by gently pushing through on the head, through the seventh cervical vertebra, or through the legs or the pelvis in the direction of the vertebral column.

Special attention should be paid to the flexibility of the trunk and to the breathing movements; these might be impaired to a greater or lesser degree by this pattern of "holding" a specific posture. The ease of movement of the shoulderblade and the clavicle should be ascertained so that the underlying ribs can more readily participate in the breathing movements. Some ribs might move unsatisfactorily during breathing or perhaps not at all. This problem can be helped during the breathing-out by means of very gentle push on the ribs, in and down, in order to elicit the expansion during the breathing-in.

All these are done very gently, and any progress or achievement should be given the teacher's encouragement. Any achievement, however small, may be a boost to the pupil's morale, but no claim is made that Functional Integration is a way to treat the emotional aspect of the problem. Nor should the teacher promise the pupil or the family that the scoliosis will be straightened out. What can be achieved is an improvement in functions related to the scoliosis. With an adult pupil, it is unlikely that more could be achieved.

On the other hand, there are cases in which complete recovery or almost complete recovery is achieved. S. T., a fourteen-year-old girl, came with her mother, with the consent of the attending physician, to consult me and find out whether Functional Integration could do something for her. She was found to have a scoliosis of fifteen degrees, and her mother told me that it was proposed that S. T. wear a so-called Milwaukee brace (an orthopedic device that must be worn most of the time). Usually it is prescribed for teenagers with pronounced scoliosis, to be worn until the growth process in the bones is completed. S. T.'s parents considered this to be too severe a measure, and they therefore were seeking alternative ways of dealing with the problem.

Asking various questions, I learned that S. T. had undergone an appendectomy two years earlier. During the initial exploratory session, I found that S. T.'s abdominal muscles on the right side were extremely tense. I asked her whether after this operation she had refrained from doing certain movements. She answered, "Yes, of course!" She had refrained from running and climbing upstairs, which were not really comfortable. The entire event had had quite an impact on her, as was easily understood when hearing her relate the story.

The protective pattern involving the right-side abdominal muscles was quite easily discarded, since S. T. became aware of what she had been doing unconsciously. Her breathing improved, especially on her right side, where it had been quite hampered. It took S. T. three sessions to recover the flexibility in the movements of her spine, and the movement-patterns involving the trunk became symmetrical.

4. General Hypertonicity

In order to have at least an inkling of what hypertonicity is, the reader could do the following: Press the elbows to the sides of the chest, so that the armpits are tightly closed, keep the chin tucked in towards the throat, squeeze the buttocks, keep the knees tightly together, tighten the stomach muscles, and try to walk. Add to all this a little bit of what one might do to show off one's power, and then you are quite near to the prototype of a person with general hypertonicity, in regard to muscular effort and impediment to easy movement. If the lack of conscious control over this state of affairs is included in the picture, then you are even nearer to the prototype. While you can stop all this at will, a hypertonic person will need help to demonstrate what the alternatives are in decreasing muscular tonus.

During the very first explorations, one can already sense the rigidity of most of this person's muscles. The movements that the teacher explores will be felt to be produced against the background of an already existing and continuous effort. Moving a limb may remind the teacher of what one feels while stirring a dense and sticky liquid. Such a state of affairs might be found in a person who is in a sense athletic, but not very efficient in movement—the person might be more attentive to muscular strength than to agility.

At the other end of the range of possibilities is the elderly person who has suffered quite a few traumatic experiences in life, and who is afraid of faltering or slipping while walking; there may even be problems with equilibrium.

It is necessary for such a person to realize that movements can be done with ease and quickness and, up to a certain point, with security, and that this ease is needed for better functioning. The teacher has to explore the basic neuro-motor functions and to make particular use of integrating manipulons that emphasize nimbleness and agility of movement.

For example, after having clarified the range of movement in bringing the elbow up over the head and back down, one can move the elbow away from the stomach into extension of the shoulder joint *slowly* and come back *fast*. One can restrict oneself here to a small and secure portion of the range of movement, such as the one nearer to the stomach, and repeat the movements quickly a few times, back and forth. Other similarly done manipulons may remove part of the "stickiness" of this person's movements, since the possibility of making the movements safely may be rediscovered. This will come with a change in the level of control.

A similar approach might be to utilize repetitive oscillatory movements, as described in chapter 7. Reducing the damping forces is then equivalent to reducing the tonus of various muscles, which is a step in the re-education of the pupil's neuromotor system.

The following case history will show how hypertonicity might evolve into a major problem and how it can be abated: N. O., a slim woman in her late thirties who was married and the mother of a child, had, a year before she came to see me, undergone a major surgical intervention in the left pelvic bone. The purpose of the surgery, she told me, was to correct a congenital malformation in her left hip joint. She had been suffering a great deal of pain in this hip joint for some time before the operation. She seemed to me quite depressed, probably because of the fact that a year after the operation she still had pains and restriction of movement in the left hip joint, as well as pain in the small of the back.

The muscles all over her body showed themselves to be tense and stringy. By the second session, the movements in the limbs were eased a bit, and the movement of the left leg in particular had become easier and less painful. She also learned how to let herself breathe with the involvement of the ribs, which meant of course giving up the superfluous tonus in the abdominal muscles. The easy breathing movements established themselves only after the head and neck became capable of easy movements. The sudden increase in oxygen supply caused her, when she stood up, to feel dizzy for a few seconds, proving how deficient her breathing had been before. Gradually the general tonus of her muscles decreased, her overall feeling improved radically, and the pain subsided within four or five sessions. Her walking movements became easy, flexible, and full of vitality. The image she had of herself as someone with a crippled body changed into the image of a person acting with self-confidence and efficiency.

5. Low Back Pain

As with any of the neuro-motor deficiencies, low back pain may be linked to structural, functional, emotional, traumatic, or neurological problems. By way of Functional Integration one can approach low back pain to the degree that it involves levels of control. It may well be that this aspect is the primary one, and then such help can be quite significant.

The CNS, with its motor, effector system, reacts to pain and discomfort by tensing up, apparently for protection. This is of course done by instinct, or in other words, it is low-level controlled. The tendency to protect serves a biological purpose: to counteract any possible endangering movement. On the other hand, an uncontrolled muscular spasm might in itself be a source of pain and discomfort. The problem thus becomes amplified, sometimes, and the system is caught up in a vicious circle of pain–spasm–more pain–more spasm.

In order to escape this vicious circle, it is necessary to change the spastic reaction of the CNS. This could be done by involving a different level of control, obviously a higher and more conscious one. The instinct itself seems sometimes to be self-defeating. It is perhaps advisable to calm down the instinctive reaction and then propose a different one, as in the following example:

The pupil is asked to lie on one side, choosing whichever seems to be the more comfortable (the fetus position, session 1). One would probably lie on the side that bothers one less. Let us suppose that the pupil lies on the left side with the knees bent at right angles to the stomach. The teacher starts by substituting for the effort of the extensors of the back on the right side, mainly in the lumbar region, by bringing the chest and the pelvis nearer to each other (confining manipulon). The direction of the push or the locations of the hands have to be adjusted and changed if necessary. In order to provide the system with the feeling that it can rely on the support provided by the teacher's hands, the smallest push and the most minute movement may be sufficient. The teacher should be aware of the fact that communication is being carried out with a low-level part of the CNS. Any change in the tonus of these muscles may be barely perceptible.

When the teacher senses that a change in tonicity is occurring, the example may be utilized for various movement-patterns involving the muscles. This of course has to be done with the utmost gentleness and very slowly, in order not to produce the slightest feeling of insecurity or of "danger." No direct and bilateral flexion or extension of the back that might involve the troubled extensors in their primary functions should be attempted; attention will instead be shifted to their antagonists.

Next, the teacher sits behind the pupil, who is still in the former position. With the right hand, the teacher pushes the right side of the pupil's pelvis in the direction of the thigh, while the left hand holds the lower rib cage to prevent it from participating in this movement. In this manner a slight flexion of the right side of the pelvis is produced with only a suggestion of a twist. The teacher has to ascertain, by asking the pupil, if this movement is causing any pain.

After a few repetitions, the teacher will use the left hand to push the upper part of the chest forward, pushing behind the right shoulder while restraining the lower part of the chest with the right hand, as had been done before by the left. This will complete the image of a flexion of the trunk. It will not provoke the system to resist the movement, since attention is drawn more to the front side. On the other hand, this last manipulon hints a twist in the upper part of the right trunk that will soon be used all along the length of the trunk.

When the teacher feels that the pupil can allow the right shoulder and the upper part of the thorax to move forward and leave the lower part behind, in other words, that the possibility of such a twist can be acknowledged by the pupil, the right hand can be shifted from the lower ribs to the pelvis, in front of the right greater trochanter. With the right hand, the pelvis is held in place while the right shoulder is pushed slightly forward as before. Eventually, the right hand may be used for the coming-back movement, so that pushing the shoulder forward alternates with pulling the pelvis back.

After a few repetitions, the simultaneous movement of the shoulder forward and the pelvis back may be possible. This can be summed up by a confining manipulon that not only emphasizes the twist of the trunk, but also the increased distance between the shoulder and the hip joint. A more specific change is likely to occur in the small ribs on the right side, where more participation in the breathing movements may be noticed. All of these movements are small, gentle, and never fast.

The spasm in the extensors of the back is associated with spasm in the extensors of the thigh (the glutei muscles). This linkage is easily understood when one considers patterns of movement in which both groups of muscles are working together, as in bending forward and lifting something off the floor. The synergism of the glutei and the extensors of the back is well established. Consequently, some clarification of the patterns involving the use of the hip joint would be useful.

With the pupil in the same position as before, the teacher sits facing the pupil's knees. The pupil's thighs are positioned at right angles to the spine, and the lower legs at right angles to the thighs. The teacher's left hand supports the pupil's right leg near the ankle from underneath and lifts it slightly, while the right knee is continuously supported by the left one (fig. 31). In fact, this will produce a rotation of the right thigh around itself. Chances are that the teacher will feel the pupil involuntarily "helping" in this lifting of the ankle, and when the leg is allowed to descend, the lower leg may simply hang there, frozen in the air. The muscle which is instrumental in producing this less-than-conscious reaction is easily found. By placing the right hand in the area between the greater trochanter and the iliac crest, the teacher feels this muscle tensing up (the gluteus medius muscle). The pupil could then be asked to stop this contraction: "Leave the heel alone! Let it fall down!" Only then

Fig. 31

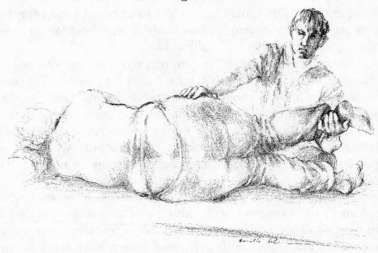

will the muscle be relaxed, but even so it might start to tense all over again with the teacher's next lift of the leg.

The teacher may notice that, concomitant with this tensing up of the gluteus medius, the muscles on the right side connecting the pelvis and the chest may tense up as well. There are of course mechanical reasons for this. If the pelvis has to hold the leg up in the air, it has to anchor itself to the rest of the body (to the chest). This is the same synergism mentioned earlier, which acts under low-level control. One way of clarifying this situation and of presenting possible alternatives is to introduce other manipulons. They should stop the synergism and raise the level of control. The use of a distal movement, the most distal part being verbally indicated, and the simultaneous monitoring of the working muscle by the teacher's touch, are conducive to raising the level of control as well.

When the tensing up of the gluteus medius is quite prominent, it is useful to place the pupil's right hand there for monitoring the activity of the muscle. The pupil may perceive the bulging up of this muscle, even when the teacher only barely touches the ankle, as if starting to lift it. The insight that the pupil may gain from this can help to gain control around the hip joint without difficulty. Using the *sense of touch as feedback*, the pupil might eventually discover and perceive the proprioceptive information from this area that was previously blurred.

With this clarification, the anchoring of the pelvis to the chest may also cease, which means refined control over the muscles of the small of the back. This can be important, considering the fact that the extensors of the back are less accessible to conscious control. The discontinuation of the anchoring of the pelvis also frees the ribs to participate more fully in breathing (see the paragraph on breathing in chapter 5). It should be mentioned in this regard that the extensors of the back cover the ribs from the outside and, when they are in spasm, they prevent the ribs from flaring out and thus interfere with breathing. On the other hand, the improved breathing movements can inhibit these extensors from tensing up.

One of the sessions to be done in a case of lower back pain, perhaps the second or the third in order, is session 6, which is done in the kneeling position.

The simultaneous spasm of the flexors and the extensors of the trunk presses the vertebrae towards each other. This pressure may be several times the pressure usually produced when the body is erect. Increased pressure of the vertebrae against each other occurs normally when a heavy object is lifted or when sudden forceful movements are made, such as jumping, running, and the like. These are normally done only for a short while. On the other hand, if such increased pressure goes on uninterruptedly, it may not be withstood by the intervertebral disks. It is a known fact that lower back pain and lumbar intervertebral disk damage are interrelated. In some cases it is believed that one causes the other.

The lower lumbar region is a notorious problem area. Increased pressure impacts the disks, so that at some places they may protrude (herniated disks) and touch the nerve rootlets of the sciatic nerve. These nerve rootlets stem from the spinal cord and emerge between the vertebrae. A protruding disk is then very near such a rootlet. Different degrees of damage inflicted on these nerve rootlets may produce any number of conditions in the leg, such as numbness, intense pain, and impairment in movement.

In such a case, manipulons similar to those outlined can be utilized, but they must be much more gentle and refined, and progress will probably be slower. The restrictions related to cases having a medical aspect, as stated at the beginning of the present chapter, apply all the more in these cases. One has to consider that the outer layers of a nerve or perhaps the nerve itself may be irritated or damaged to some degree, and even small movements, in which the irritating agents touch the irritated place, may increase the pain. It is important to help the pupil to discover static positions in which the pain is diminished, so that there is a possibility for the irritated places to heal. The pupil should be advised not to initiate pain-producing movements or exercises, since this only worsens the irritation.

It so happens that an intervertebral disk, even herniated, still retains some of its elasticity, so that diminished pressure among the neighboring vertebrae can bring about the retraction of the protruding part. The important point is that the pupil learn to get rid of the spasm by gaining better control over certain muscles, and this diminishes the probability of the spastic pattern returning.

In connection with lower back pain, it is sometimes said that a vertebra is "out of place." The spasm of the back muscles holds the vertebra out of position and, by increasing the friction, prevents an easy return to its place. From a functional-dynamical point of view, there is no such thing as a precisely determined and fixed position of two neighboring vertebrae, one relative to the other. Rather, there is a continuum of possible relative positions in accordance with the potential movements that these vertebrae can engage in. The various movements of the spinal column, such as flexion, extension, side bend or twist, are always the total sum of the minute movements occurring between any pair of neighboring vertebrae. The less the vertebrae are pressed towards each other, the easier these movements will be. In other words, the best condition is for the back muscles to be without excessive tonus. It is reasonable to assume—and this is what really happens in practice—that with the diminution of this tonus, a displaced vertebra will easily regain its position during the various movements of the vertebral column occurring in normal, easy circumstances.

6. Neuro-Motor Impairment

The intention here is not to deal extensively with the problem of rehabilitating the neurologically impaired. On the other hand, a review is needed of the ways of approaching these problems from the viewpoint of Functional Integration, which can help in a great number of such cases in spite of the immense diversity of problems.

Cases of CNS damage are usually grouped by the disease, process, or event that is considered to have caused the damage, such as cerebral palsy (CP), polio, stroke, injuries involving the central or peripheral nervous system, operations involving the nervous system, and many more.

As long as learning ability is still preserved, that is to say, as long as the CNS has the ability to change and to improve its functions, there is a possibility of assisting such a learning process.

As a starting point, the state of the person's faculties should be observed. The strategy should be to proceed gradually from this point, rather than to aim towards any final result, which might not be achievable at all. Only when the damage is really minor can one expect the person to reach complete rehabilitation. There will be some cases in which significant improvement can be achieved and others in which the improvement is slow and small.

The real importance of such a learning process is not the

achievement of the ultimate goal, but the fact that new options for learning and improvement are being opened for the person.

A person who has some functions impaired or destroyed will be in what is called a state of regression. This means that the CNS and the carrying-out and sensing parts of the system are functioning, but the affected parts are working as they once worked at a certain earlier stage of development. For example, one who is impaired in many functions, neuro-motor or other, is still breathing, can swallow and cough, may move the head and eyes, and move the limbs in a more or less differentiated way. In a state such as this, it is as if one had regressed to an earlier stage of development, at least insofar as it concerns the affected part of the system.

If the impairment is a consequence of what happened in adult life, a stroke or the like, then the faculties acquired later in life might suffer more than the inherited ones, or those that had been acquired earlier in life and are therefore more deeply "ingrained" in the system. If, for example, there is partial impairment in the functions of one of the hands, then the functions still remaining might be undifferentiated, gross movements, while the differentiated and refined movements of the fingers might be more affected.

A similar thing will happen with more complex brain functions as well. If, for example, the person knew many languages and suffered brain damage affecting the language faculty, then it may be the native tongue rather than any of the acquired foreign languages that is still intact.

If the impairment is congenital, as in CP, then the impeded learning processes relative to the normal stages of development will be similar to those of an earlier stage, at least insofar as the affected functions are concerned.

There is still another important facet of regression that is central to the literal meaning of the term, namely, that when one experiences the shock of realizing that abilities one could once count on are no longer extant, one restricts oneself to only those patterns of action that seem to be the safest and best known—those that have been learned earlier in life. Sometimes this means that the person gives up certain patterns that were not at all affected.

B. L., a young man in his late twenties, had been stricken by a viral disease that produced minor damage in the CNS in the first year of his life. As a result, he had a paresis (a partial paralysis) on the right side. The right leg and right foot had not attained their full development; they were shorter and smaller than the left leg and foot. He wouldn't stretch out his knee completely, and he had a slight limp. The right arm and right hand, both appreciably smaller than the left ones, seemed as if paralyzed—they were held in a rigid way close to the body with the elbow slightly bent and the wrist constantly flexed. He didn't use the right hand and arm at all, except for holding light objects between the upper arm and the body. B. L. appeared to be a very intelligent person, and other faculties seemed to be unaffected.

The most prominent malfunction discovered during my first explorations was the rigidity of B. L.'s right shoulder, which didn't allow the elbow to change the position in which it was continuously held. Only after clarifying the possibilities for easier movement in the trunk and the chest could the right shoulder blade become a little more movable. I had to return from time to time to the movements of the trunk and especially to the breathing movements, in order to assure the assimilation of the element of increased movability.

Subsequently, when the shoulderblade's movability allowed this, I took the elbow forward, so that I could ultimately put the back of the right hand near the left cheek. First, I assisted with a forward movement of the head. When he first felt the touch of the hand on the face, he allowed a slight rolling of the right forearm around itself, so that ultimately the palm of the hand could touch below the chin (supination of the forearm).

With both my hands I held his right hand and his head together as one unit and rotated them in both directions (a non-differentiated movement). Now I could release his head (B. L.

was lying on his back) and do a similar circular movement with the arm, which I was holding by the elbow and wrist (differentiated movement). Again I brought the hand towards his face, first the back of the hand towards the left cheek as before, and then again, through supination, which was easier this time, the palm of the hand. Now I held the wrist in place on his cheek, and with my other hand I turned his head a little bit to the left and then a little bit to the right, so that his fingers were brushing different places on his face. I made these movements with the utmost gentleness, and this induced B. L. to relax his fingers so that they would not hurt his face.

Gradually I changed over, leaving the head stationary while moving the hand left and right (relative conjugate movements). It turned out in this way that his right hand could reach for many more places on the face without having to be helped with the movements of the head.

When I returned the hand for a moment to the place he had been holding it all the time and began to bring it to his face once more, the rigidity reappeared. Still, I brought his hand back to his face, helping, as in the beginning, by moving the shoulder-blade. Now I asked B. L. to allow me to take his hand away from his face and to allow it to return *immediately* to the face. After a few trials, this big movement in the shoulder joint with the involvement of the scapula became easier, with somewhat of an increased range.

B. L. admitted afterwards that this had been the first time he had ever felt the touch of his right hand on his face.

One can see to what early stages of development one has to revert (early infancy) in order to validly reconstruct various functions. It should also be pointed out that the touching of hand to face not only has the significance of a primary, primitive movement that is necessary at a certain stage of development, but that it also provides an intimacy with oneself that feels comfortable, like being "at home."

Another relevant fact is that the inability to move a distal part, such as the hand, causes the person to make efforts in the respective proximal part. This effort may be possible, but at the same time it is totally inefficient from the point of view of the initial intention. Moreover, these proximal efforts, with their resulting rigidity, both blur and obstruct the discovery of possible differentiations in the weaker distal muscles. This has special importance where the envisaged patterns were never present and have to be created and then incorporated into the movement-patterns of the pupil. From the start, one is not able to imagine or to represent such a pattern. This had been the case with B. L., who couldn't imagine what it was to produce a differentiated action with his right hand or fingers.

In order to allow this kind of discovery in a playful way, as it usually occurs in the child's course of development, one has to help this person to reduce the constant proximal effort greatly, as a necessary preparatory stage.

A situation of this kind is quite often encountered in cases of neuro-motor impairment. Usually, the integration of this giving-up of the proximal effort is not easily attained. It actually calls for a change of the person's *attitude toward his intention to act.* In other words, the person must acknowledge the fact that various patterns of action, which are unclear, blurred, or perhaps even nonexistent in his experience—such as using fingers independently for various actions, or opposition of the thumb and the like—have to be searched for *playfully* and *with minute efforts,* eliminating bigger efforts which obliterate the more refined discrimination that is needed for programming more refined movements (the Weber-Fechner Law). Mere will power directed towards achieving the goal, which is usually associated with muscular effort, thus obstructs the learning process and should be given up.

The way in which the easy movability in the wrist was achieved, after having been constantly in a rigid, flexed state, underlines an important principle. The fact that the extensors of the wrist and of the fingers were continuously inactive deprived the flexors of any inhibition (remember the reciprocal inhibition of antagonists). The flexors, working continuously,

were consequently short and rigid. Another aspect of this situation was that the continuous activation of the flexors provided
continuous inhibition of the extensors. This prevented B. L.
from utilizing whatever slight ability he might have had to
activate them. As mentioned before, I rolled B. L.'s right forearm around itself while his hand was touching the head, and in
this way I was circumventing the distorted antagonism between the flexors and the extensors of the wrist. On the other
hand, the very unusual but very dramatic sensation of the hand
and face touching each other provided a new context in which
he could relate the possible extension of the wrist.

An additional element involved here was that the supination
of the forearm—starting in the position in which the back of the
hand touched the cheek when done with flexed wrist and
fingers—would have pressed the fingers directly into the cheek
uncomfortably. The instinctive defense against such a possibility, which is of course low-level controlled, was thus used for a
positive and constructive purpose (this defense was a slight
extension of the wrist and the fingers in order to avoid scratching the face). The relaxation of the flexors stopped the inhibition
of the extensors, or at least diminished it, and this opened the
way for the possible use of the extensors.

The pronation and supination of the forearm was used as a
way of changing the context of the flexion-extension in other
situations as well. B. L. was lying on his stomach with his face
towards the left and his right hand somehow alongside the
body. After having ascertained that the right shoulder could be
lifted up from the table, I elevated his right elbow slightly with
one of my hands and with the other I rolled his right forearm
back and forth over his pelvis. Eventually I succeeded, without
force, in putting his forearm across his back at the level of the
belt, and then continued "playing" with the pronation-supina-
tion of the forearm, while checking the possibility of extension-
flexion movements in the wrist. By doing this, B. L.'s fingers
became relaxed and easily pliable.

When I slipped B. L.'s right hand into his back trouser pocket, the palm alternately facing this way and the other, it was a revelation to him. Once the giving-up of the spasticity established itself, a similar way of checking could be tried out with the hand in front of the body.

In the meanwhile, I had to deal with still another aspect of B. L.'s inefficient way of organizing himself. Since certain joints had been held in a slightly flexed position continuously (the knees, the hip joints, and the right elbow), the efficient use of the skeleton had not developed clearly enough (see chapter 5). The feeling that forces could be allowed to transmit themselves through the skeleton was not familiar enough to B. L.—neither in his legs, as it would be in standing, nor in his right arm, as it would be in using the arm to push or to support his body. Moreover, the right elbow joint seemed to be structurally deficient and it appeared that complete extension of the elbow joint was therefore impossible. This was a striking example of a deficient structural development that related to functional deficiency.

A state of deteriorated reciprocal antagonism such as existed in the flexion-extension of the wrist appeared also in the flexion-extension of the right elbow in relation to the biceps and triceps muscles.

Usually one learns efficient use of the skeleton quite early in life, together with the first assumption of the erect posture and with the first attempts at pushing something away. It was now necessary to provide B. L. with this sensation by slight pushes through the feet, while he was lying on his back, comparing right and left sides as we proceeded. With the right arm B. L. had more difficulty, not only because of the structural deficiency in the elbow. For example, while sitting facing him, I asked him to lean slightly forward and push me with his right hand, which I held with my two hands. He did the opposite: he leaned back slightly and pulled me towards himself. It was not that he didn't understand what he was supposed to do; with his left hand he could do exactly what he was expected to do. The *determination to make an effort* brought him to use his flexors instead of his extensors. The solution was, as always, to give up the intention of doing something with effort. To promote this, I held his right hand in front of him with my hands while he was bent slightly forward, and I told him that I would slowly try to come nearer to him and the only thing he had to do was to see if he could, without effort, keep the distance as it was. This idea seemed to be incorporated more easily in B. L.'s image of achievement, and he gradually learned how to use his triceps and inhibit the flexion of his elbow; in other words, to extend his arm as an intentional action.

Subsequently, B. L. discovered that with a slight extension of the elbow, the effort in the triceps was diminished, allowing him to lean forward and push more efficiently. The only muscles that still had to make an effort—and this did not present any problem—were the muscles of the trunk. Gradually, more patterns involving skeletal alignment established themselves as efficient and easy.

I put a broomstick in B. L.'s hands and, while he lay on his back with the stick across his stomach, I asked him to lift the stick above his head. This was done in two ways: one, with the elbows on the table on both sides of the body, and the other with the elbows lifted. I asked him to do no more with his good left hand than he was doing with his right hand, so that the movement would be symmetrical. In this way, I diverted his attention from wanting to reach out more with the left hand, so that he began consciously monitoring what he was doing, comparing the left and the right hands. The result was that the extension of the right arm improved.

More variations were added to this, such as moving one arm ahead of the other, moving both arms simultaneously in opposite directions, and moving the stick left and right at different levels.

The motor and sensory link between both hands and arms provided by the stick, as well as the participation of both arms in the same movement pattern, were helping to establish the image of the right arm in action.

I used the same stick to obtain a refinement of the actions of the palm and fingers: with B. L. sitting and holding the stick across his lap with both hands, I asked him to relax the grip of one hand very slightly, so that the other could slide the stick through the curve of the fingers a little bit. Then the first hand had to grip again and slide the stick through the second, which then released its grip slightly, the stick moving back to the same side as before. Doing this alternately with both hands, the stick was moved a few inches to one side and then to the other. Playing in this manner with the stick, each hand had to grip and release alternately without making a noticeable movement with the fingers. At the same time, both fists were moving nearer and farther from each other while alternately sliding and grasping the stick.

It should be pointed out that B. L. was not asked to make what might be called an abstract movement but rather reality-related actions.

The stick had a few other uses as well. B. L. sat with the stick propped up in a vertical position between his knees, and his hands "climbed up" the stick a few steps and back down again. Or, holding the stick horizontally with both hands in front of himself, B. L. lifted it up and put it behind his neck. Another one was to take the stick in one hand—starting with the left— and to bring it overhead so that it could touch the back in a diagonal way, and then reach behind and take hold of it with the other hand, near the pelvis. With both hands gripping the stick in this way, he shifted the stick so that it slid up and down or left and right on his back.

With a shorter and thinner stick (about half an inch in diameter) in his right hand, B. L. was asked to point with it in different directions, touch different places with it, or draw straight lines or circles with it. In this way he was trying out voluntary movements with his wrist.

Along the same line of thinking, I put a tube of cardboard, one inch in diameter, in B. L.'s right hand. He had to look through it at different objects that were pointed out to him. This necessitated a further degree of refinement and control, first, to succeed in not hurting his eye with the tube and, secondly, to make a finer adjustment while directing the tube at a specific point.

B. L. learned how to interlace the fingers of both hands and move them above the head towards his neck. In this position, the movements of the elbows towards each other and away from each other could be easily checked and attempted.

Only a part of what was done with B. L. has been described here, mainly in order to illustrate certain points of principle. In fact, B. L. had some twenty sessions spread out over a period of two years, but grouped in three intensive, short periods. His walking became much more balanced and straight and, when he didn't hurry, his limp was almost imperceptible. Both shoulders became broad and quite symmetrical and his right arm hung down almost freely. The use of the right hand appeared to be firmly established, and he went on playing with it and trying out more possibilities along the lines developed during our sessions. It is apparent from the above descriptions that B. L. was asked to produce quite a few movements by himself. This was, indeed, the case, but my help was essential with many movements, at least in the beginning, and help was offered by way of appropriate manipulons.

One last fact worth mentioning is that B. L.'s right elbow could be extended significantly more as the sessions progressed than in the beginning. This proves the possibility of improving a structural deficiency by improving the function. The structural distortion was probably related more to soft tissues than to the bones, and these adapted themselves to the restricted functioning of the joint. With the change of the functions, the soft tissues (cartilages and interstitial tissues) adapted themselves to allow an increased range of movement in the joint.

Finally, B. L. brought me a letter of thanks written with his right hand, the same hand that for so many years had been only a useless appendage of his body.

From among the myriad problems to be found in the vast area of neurological impairment, I want to single out two for a few additional comments, namely, *spasticity* and *uncontrolled movements.*

Spasticity is the simultaneous activation of an antagonistic pair of muscles that is low-level controlled. Often, the particular lower level involved is what in neuro-physiology is called the extrapyramidal system. Sometimes, the possibility of gaining upper-level control is very slight, and with some cases it seems impossible to attain. It sometimes happens that spasticity is diminished for a while, but then a slight irritation of one of the involved muscles (or a seemingly unrelated irritation) will trigger the spasticity again, bringing it back in its full vigor. If one can succeed in controlling the spastic reaction by stopping or at least delaying it, it indicates that one has succeeded in using the cortico-spinal tract and can bypass the extrapyramidal tract, but only sporadically. However, this also means that optimal situations should be sought that enable one to do this again and again. The channel connecting the cortex with the so-called common pathway will be used repeatedly and "trodden out," thus increasing the probability of having its function established.

The optimal situations described above will certainly be different with different cases, but often one can reach them by doing movements different from the movements involving the spastic pair of antagonists, as, for instance, turning the lower leg around itself, in the case of spasticity that forces the knee to be straight (the first part of schematic session 5).

It should be clear that where there is more serious damage of the CNS, the handling of spasticity and other functional disturbances can be very difficult indeed.

It seems sometimes that the spastic straightening out of the leg is totally unrelated to the purposes or functions for which the leg is normally straightened out (reaching out for support or stepping on the leg by extending it, followed by the appropriate use of the skeleton the moment such support is felt).

In the normal functioning of the leg, the sense of touch on the soles of the foot (the first part of the leg to contact the floor)

plays an obvious role. The sense of touch on the sole of the foot
is an important ingredient in the pattern of standing or walking
in an efficient way. This linkage of the sense of touch with
antigravitational patterns is probably established very early,
perhaps even phylogenetically. In case of spasticity of one or
both legs, this role is somehow occluded. There is a way of
isolating this element from the antigravitational concerns of the
pupil's system by having the pupil lie down on the work table
and creating what could be called an artificial floor.

The pupil lies on the back, with legs extended and with the
soles of the feet slightly over-reaching the edge of the table (the
ankles are best supported by a small soft roller). The teacher sits
by the feet, and, with a smooth, flat piece of board made of
wood, thick cardboard, or even styrofoam and slightly larger
than the sole of the foot itself, gently touches various places on
the sole of the foot. It is best to start with the most distal part
of the foot, which in the pupil's kinesthetic sensation, is the
small toe on the outside. Barely moving it, the teacher touches
it with the board, moving towards its plantar surface and back,
and gradually involving the fourth toe also. While rotating towards the plantar surface, the board may leave the very tip of
the toe (or of the two last toes), and when returning it touches
the tips again.

It might happen, when the toes are bent upwards or dor-
siflexed (this is common), that this playful action of giving a hint
of some support and having it slowly withdrawn will elicit a
special reaction: namely, the toe (or toes) will descend with the
receding "floor," following it in order not to lose touch. This
very ancient way of reacting is, in a sense, totally new in the
pupil's experience, since it has never been enacted (or at least,
not recently). It also has the quality of being a most gentle
movement in a limb that has experienced only violent movement and large effort.

This way of touching and "teasing" gradually involves all the
toes, and while turning towards the plantar surface, it involves

the entire sole of the foot. Done with dexterity, this artificial floor will also elicit flexion in the ankle and the eversion of the foot. In other words, the leg prepares itself for standing, being stimulated by something that is sensed as a floor.

When the pupil subsequently assumes an upright position, this old-new ingredient of the antigravitational patterns will have a chance to be implemented.

It should be pointed out that the use of an artificial floor briefly described here proceeds quite slowly. If it is also done on the other foot, and then on both together, it will require a complete session.

Uncontrolled movements can be related to a variety of neurological disorders. There are diffent kinds of uncontrolled movements, such as tremors of various kinds, clonic movements that are an uncontrolled alternation of flexion and extension, or athetotic movements, the latter being disordered movements that occur mainly in the limbs, the head, and the face, seemingly without any purpose whatsoever.

As with spasticity, uncontrolled movements involve an exclusion of the cortico-spinal tract, and one of the ways of bringing the cortex into having its say once again is to find areas or contexts in which intentional action can make use of the motor system to circumvent the extrapyramidal system. One has to discover and propose to the pupil intentional patterns of action carried out by the same parts of the body that produce the uncontrolled movements. These patterns may in some ways be similar to one of the uncontrolled movements, but they should be different in at least one of their parameters. For instance, one goes along with the pupil's movement and changes its velocity, making it slower, for example, and thus blunting a possible jerkiness of the movement; or one does a slow rhythmical movement instead of an unrhythmical one, or changes the direction slightly.

All these actions might arouse the "interest" of the cortex (the somato-sensory cortex and the intentional cortex) and provide the necessary ingredients for cortical control and programming.

It sometimes suffices to deal with a small part of the motor system, such as one hand, or one particular movement of the hand, and the calming-down process will spread out over other parts of the body and other uncontrolled movements will calm down as well. In this way use is made of the property the CNS has of *equalizing the level of excitation* in its various parts.

The reader has probably noticed that a certain strategy keeps recurring, especially in dealing with neuro-motor impairment: namely, the strategy of providing the pupil with the necessary or lacking component for generating a pattern of action that is deficient or inexistent. Sometimes such a component is nothing other than a certain element within the CNS reaction pattern that is already ingrained in the system. The situation has to be set up so that this reaction is elicited. In other cases, the component is directly provided by the teacher as an auxiliary movement, or as an inhibiting part of a certain ongoing pattern, or as sensory information that is bound to become part of the ultimately emerging pattern.

The new patterns should be conducive to intentional actions, (upper-level controlled) and as such, should bypass the reflexive or other low-level controlled mechanisms.

Notwithstanding certain generalizations concerning the technique that the reader has encountered in this chapter, it should be emphasized again that the main attribute of Functional Integration is the unpreconceived approach of the teacher to every pupil. General directives should not deter the teacher from having constantly in mind the individual traits and the special needs of the pupil.

11. Additional Do's and Don'ts for a Future Practitioner

The first session in a series will usually start with an interview of the pupil. The pupil describes complaints or problems, if any; the teacher will of course ask how long these problems have continued and what has been done about them up until now. It should be made clear if there has been any medical treatment and whether this treatment is still continuing. Any information about surgery or major injuries in the past may also be of relevance. In short, the teacher has to verify that this is by no means a clinical case, but that the pupil is a healthy person from the medical point of view. A person who is under current medical supervision or who is undergoing medical treatment should definitely not be accepted as a pupil, unless the attending physician consents.

It should be explained beforehand that the pupil is not going to receive a "treatment" and should not expect any "cure." On the other hand, the pupil should be told to expect to learn something about behaviors, motor patterns, and ways of moving with more efficiency and comfort. The teacher should inform the pupil that any changes that may happen will not be a direct result of the sessions (which are in fact lessons), but will be a result of the insights gained during these lessons and that these insights may help create behaviors different from the habitual ones.

After a short verbal interchange of this kind, one can begin with the first session. Supposedly, the teacher already has an idea of how to start the session and in which position, according to what is already known about the person, including what has been observed visually.

The pupil remains clothed. The clothing should preferably be loose and soft. Only the shoes are taken off, in order to make lying on the table more comfortable. This point is important, because every session should proceed in an atmosphere of normal communicative interaction between two people. One should avoid the possibility of any embarrassment as well as any association with medical examination or treatment.

Since the teacher is not yet acquainted with the pupil's degree of sensitivity, the explorations are begun in a very gentle and reserved way and in areas in which they are not likely to arouse defensive reactions, even when these seem not overtly present. The teacher should make use of any impressions about the pupil's social upbringing, status, age, and any other particular characteristics that might bear on the person's sensitivity. The pupil's gender should be taken into consideration as well. The teacher has to be aware of the social, cultural, or individual significance of one person touching another. It is well known how differently people might define the term "intimate place."

The teacher will surely not want to touch a place that the pupil might consider as intimate to some degree. Exploratory manipulons are therefore begun in places such as the back, between the shoulders (where, by the way, the exploration might be needed anyway), and then expanded in a necessary and logical fashion. On the other hand, there will be places which the teacher will strictly avoid.

The presence of a third person during the session should be allowed only with the pupil's approval.

Structural deficiencies or blemishes found by the teacher during the session should not be pointed out to the pupil, unless it is necessary for a factual clarification.

All these remarks are based on the need to produce in the pupil a feeling of confidence and security, so that the attention can be focused on the kinesthetic sensations, the first step in creating a learning situation.

In the second session, as well as in the following ones, the teacher will check to what extent the clarifications and changes have been assimilated by the pupil; in other words, one can start by checking the functions that were scrutinized in the previous sessions, this time possibly in a different position. If this is done clearly, the pupil will also become aware of the linkage between sessions and realize that each session continues something that was dealt with in the previous lesson. Such a developing insight enhances the learning experience.

The duration of a session should be kept within the limit of forty-five minutes, but one has to remember that even this amount of time may be too much for elderly persons or for a person who is in pain.

Unless there are special reasons for doing it otherwise, a day or two should be allowed between sessions. The pupil should have the time and opportunity to try out things freely, and to become used to particular changes that may have occurred.

The teacher should be the one who proposes to discontinue the series of sessions, either when the main purpose has been achieved, or when the pupil's progress is no longer significant.

We will not discuss here the legal right of one person to touch another person. On the other hand, the *moral* right to touch another person presupposes the harmlessness of this touch. In other words, one has to be absolutely sure that one will not be risking any harm to the other person. If there is the slightest doubt, one should absolutely abstain from doing anything at all. Functional Integration is supposed to teach something, and if this teaching is for any reason not likely to occur, then one should stop doing it, or even not start it at all.

Speaking of the harmlessness of touch, one should remember a slogan of the medical profession, which could apply to many other professions as well. It surely fits Functional Integration:

Primum non nocere. It means: The first principle is to do no harm.

Obviously, the gentleness of the manipulations not only makes them a teaching tool, as has already been amply demonstrated, but also assures their harmlessness. Yet, Functional Integration should be considered a powerful tool, since it can suddenly make clear to the pupil possibilities that his structure may not be ready for. A pupil with any fragility of structure, after having gained some degree of freedom of movement or an increased range of movement, should be warned not to exploit these newly achieved abilities immediately, but rather to implement them gradually.

Without intending it at all, the teacher is sometimes faced with a medical problem. The pupil may have failed to report some specific health problem in the beginning, such as a heart condition or something else, having considered this fact irrelevant to the reasons for wanting sessions of this sort. A teacher should in such a case cut off the lesson at once and not resume the sessions, until receiving the full and explicit consent of the attending physician.

The fact that the pupil might mention a doctor's diagnosis does not mean that the teacher is to come up with diagnoses. This is not simply because only members of the medical profession are entitled to make diagnoses, but also and more importantly because in doing Functional Integration the teacher is never dealing with a static situation requiring a fixed name or category, but rather with a learning process in which the relevant terms are dyadic: aware–unaware, efficient–inefficient, clear–unclear, intentional–unintentional, differentiated–nondifferentiated, habitual–nonhabitual. Each of these pairs designates the two extremes of a definite functional and dynamic dimension in the "space" of human action. Any human action *finds its place* within this multi-dimensional space, and Functional Integration makes the point that this *place* is not necessarily fixed—that with a change of place, the *quality* of the action improves.

Part V

SOME ILLUSTRATIVE
CASE HISTORIES

12. The Story of Hanoch's Return to the Flute*

> E pur, si muove!
> Galileo

A person who is thrown into a traumatic situation (physically and/or emotionally) can, in some instances, overcome it—either on his own or with any help he can get—with the one condition that he take a cool and "objective" look at himself, his actual state, and all his available options. That is what happened to Hanoch Tel-Oren, first flutist with the Jerusalem Symphony Orchestra. Hanoch Tel-Oren survived a terrorist attack on March 11, 1978, during which he lost his fourteen-year-old son and was himself seriously wounded. His story is extraordinary in two respects: his personal story with its own emotional weight and drama, and the more specific story of his subsequent rehabilitation, almost spectacularly achieved by means of the Feldenkrais method of Functional Integration. In fact, both aspects are inseparably intertwined and interdependent.

Hanoch's main injury was caused by a bullet that pierced the right arm an inch or so above the elbow, not touching the bone, but disrupting the median nerve almost completely.

The surgeons did the best they could. Blood vessels and muscles were repaired, a skin graft closed the wound (skin taken from the thigh), and the forearm was put in a cast to prevent movement in the wrist. Another intervention was to be per-

* First published in *Somatics*, vol. 2, no. 3 (1979).

formed a few weeks later, in order to join the torn ends of the median nerve. The plan was subsequently given up, since the slight movements Hanoch could produce a couple of weeks after I began working with him showed that some nerve impulses were now coming through.

When I visited Hanoch at the hospital a week after the incident, the surgeon told me that they had just managed to save his arm. As for using it—"Well, very limited hopes; anyway, he will never play the flute again, nor has he been encouraged to have any hopes of that." Hanoch himself sounded more optimistic. He said that he was waiting to be discharged from the hospital so that we could continue our work. The precarious basis of his hope was that he had undergone a series of weekly sessions in Functional Integration with me the preceding months (for the purpose of "general improvement"); moreover, he knew of another flutist who had had an injury of the left radial nerve, and who succeeded in returning to full playing capacity after working with me a year-and-a-half ago.

In the beginning of May, seven weeks after the incident, Hanoch was released from the hospital and he came to see me.

His right thumb, forefinger, and middle finger were all impaired in their functions in the severest way. He couldn't flex them at all, but when they were flexed passively he could extend them. The sensation in these fingers on the palmar and side surfaces was absent. He was holding his arm flexed, with the elbow at a right angle, the forearm supinated and the wrist straight. He was, of course, unable to pronate the forearm, and there was pain in the wrist. The motor and sensory functions subserved by the median nerve all seemed lost. Hanoch's emotional state seemed to be under control, but it was clear that he was in urgent need of a show of real progress.

There was another fact of importance: His right shoulder was tense and stiff, the neck and head held in place forcefully, with a slight increase in the already existing scoliosis of the dorsal vertebrae.

Such a state of affairs has its logic: because of the frustrating

e of impotence in such circumstances, one attempts to
come it by an excessive effort, thus compensating (although
vholly consciously) for the perceived inefficiency. Repeated
sive efforts of this kind will create altered patterns of
ment, which extend to those parts of the system that are
npaired or not impaired at all. These altered patterns of
ment will likely substitute for the former ones in the rela-
up between the action as actually performed and its kines-
representation; in other words, one might see oneself
ming a certain action, while in reality performing some-
different. (Try to move your ear, and the moment you
e you're succeeding, look in the mirror to see what grim-
ou are making instead.) Secondly, these distorted patterns
vement may crowd out the very slight possibilities that
ist of being regenerated.

iously, that was my first concern with Hanoch. By gentle
ulations I had to provide him with the sensation that he
give up a whole series of persisting efforts in the trunk and
houlder girdle. I even explained to him the obvious fact
ese extra efforts, which his situation was causing him to
did not really serve any constructive pupose. Actually, I
come back to that point now and then, until Hanoch
l to control that "instinctive" tendency to channel the
owards the bigger, proximal muscles, so altering the
efulness of the action.

tendency can be understood as an effect of the regres-
e system undergoes when suddenly thrown into a state
icted capabilities. The regression is to an earlier stage of
ual development, in this case to a stage *preceding* the
g of refined, skilled uses of hands and fingers; a stage in
differentiation of and fine control over the bigger and
al muscles was learned. Now Hanoch had to be guided
hrough that learning process, which was on the one hand
ted by the fact that Hanoch's central nervous system was
rally intact and "knew how" to generate the appropriate
t impulses if it received appropriate afferent (sensory)

feedback. On the other hand there was the critically limiting condition of the interrupted nerve fibers (axons) that were still *expected to regenerate* distally—this included both *motor* and *sensory* fibers.

Wouldn't it be possible to help Hanoch to *follow up* the regeneration of the cut motor nerve fibers by promptly sending *clear* and *differentiated* efferent (motor) impulses through these fibers? Moreover, couldn't the generation of such impulses by the conscious brain possibly stimulate and further that nerve growth? One couldn't hope for any ready made answers to these questions.

Assuming a possible regeneration of axons from the place of distal disruption to the *sites of the myoneural junctions* of the different neurons, I had to also assume that functions using muscles with their myoneural junctions *nearer* to the lesion would recover *earlier*. By that reasoning, all the *motor* functions (and their corresponding muscles) subserved by the median nerve and thus affected by the lesion were placed in a very definite *sequence* of expected recovery: (1) the pronation of the forearm (pronator teres muscle), (2) the flexion of the wrist (palmaris longus, flexor carpi radialis), (3) the flexion of the index and of the middle fingers (flexor digitorum sublimis and profundus), (4) the flexion of the thumb (flexor pollicis longus), (5) another enhancement of the pronation of the forearm (pronator quadratus), (6) abduction and opposition of the thumb, and flexion in the knuckles by the intrinsic muscles of the hand (abductor pollicis brevis, flexor pollicis brevis, opponens pollicis, lumbricales).

The sensory nerve fibers provide afferent pathways for (a) impulses from the skin towards the brain that transmit the sensations of touch, pain, and temperature; (b) impulses coming from the muscle spindles (stretch-receptors); and (c) proprioceptive impulses coming from the sense organs in the tendons and joints that transmit the kinesthetic sensations.

The recovery of the *sensory* functions could be expected to occur *later* than the motor functions for the following reasons:

the greater distance to be covered by the regenerating axons, say, up to the finger tips; a possible degeneration of the posterior nerve root (in the spinal cord); the fact that the afferent impulses have to be generated in the distally situated sense organs, so that such impulses will not be transmitted before the axon succeeds in making the connection.

Since neuro-motor functioning, and even more so, neuro-motor learning, depend on appropriate sensory feedback, Hanoch had to learn to use alternative, substitutive sensory channels as pathways for feedback, until the regular sensory channels could eventually catch up. I will return to this point later.

According to the anticipated sequence of recovery mentioned before, I directed my attention (and Hanoch's) to the pronation of the forearm. A passive movement (my initiation of the movement with the forearm in the expectation it would not meet with resistance) turned out to be hardly possible, since it was met by quite a strong opposition of the antagonist muscles.

It is a known fact that the *activation* of a certain muscle has as a concomitant the *inhibition* of its antagonist (the principle of reciprocal inhibition). This function is controlled centrally (through neural pathways coming from the brain), as well as peripherally (through connections in the "ventral horn" of the corresponding segment of the spinal cord).

In our case, the inactivity of certain muscles deprived their antagonists of inhibition, but the increased activation of these antagonists was now reciprocally blocking, by inhibition, any possible way for impulses to get to the affected muscles. We had to find the means to centrally inhibit the supinators.

The difficulty Hanoch encountered at this stage was in giving up the tension in his biceps (which was acting as a flexor of the elbow and as a strong supinator). With Hanoch lying on his back on a horizontal surface, his arms alongside the body, I put the right forearm in a vertical position (the elbow resting on the surface) and rotated it slowly and repeatedly around its axis. While doing this, I also put a little stress on the supination, and so I provided the sensation of myself performing the action of the biceps, substituting *my effort* for its effort. The moment I felt that Hanoch was allowing the movement to be done with ease, I added (simultaneously with the pronation) a slight extension of the elbow with a slight dorsiflexion in the wrist, as in turning the palm down and simultaneously pushing away with the thumb. Eventually he succeeded in letting me make that last movement without preparation, taking him "by surprise."

Another way of increasing his control over the biceps was this: Hanoch had to learn to use the brachialis muscle (without the biceps!) in slightly flexing the elbow, so that the flexion could be dissociated from the supination. There was difficulty doing this at the beginning, because of strong adhesions between the outer part of the brachialis and the scarred patch covering the site of the injury. Ultimately, this difficulty turned into an advantage, because Hanoch could use the *image* of tensing that scar towards the shoulder, and that was equivalent to activating the brachialis without the biceps or to flexing the elbow without supination.

At this point I placed his right forearm across the stomach (he was lying on his back) and, propping the thumb against the left small ribs from below, he was asked to roll the forearm up over the stomach repeatedly, by *imagining* a lifting or extending of the little finger. This movement was initiated by the corresponding extensors (extensor carpi ulnaris, extensor digiti minimi), but it evoked the pronator as a synergist, and gradually the image of lifting the small finger changed into the image of pronating the forearm. Ultimately (two weeks after we began to work), the pronation started to become a reality. The first clear step forward had been taken.

Meanwhile, we had already started to deal with functions expected subsequently. The movements in the wrist joint were somewhat painful (probably because it had had to be immobilized during the first part of the hospitalization period), and so these were approached very gradually and carefully. Eventually that sensitivity in the wrist subsided and by then the active movements in that joint were already implemented.

The flexion of the index and middle fingers had to be prepared (along the same lines of thinking) by the increased control and relaxation of the antagonist extensors. I will mention only some of the work done in this area. Having Hanoch's right arm supported horizontally (except wrist and fingers, which were dangling down) and to some degree flexed by gravity, I lightly tapped every finger with one of my fingers from below in an upward direction, until he succeeded in letting it fall back and not keeping it extended.

A more differentiated control over the extensors of the fingers was achieved by having Hanoch lie on his stomach with his right hand alongside the body (palm upward). He was now asked to apply his fingernails with a little pressure to the surface on which he was lying (this was done by the extensors). I checked every finger separately until he had them all pressed down. Now he was asked to allow each finger in turn to be lifted easily by me, but without ceasing the pressure with the nails of the other fingers. Meanwhile I checked all the fingers, and, by focusing his attention, Hanoch learned to control and to coordinate this movement. After some work of this kind, I could detect a little more tonus in the flexors, and gradually Hanoch could produce the flexion, although not yet with the distal phalanges of the index finger and the thumb.

The adduction of the thumb (the movement of bringing it nearer to the index finger) was possible, but quite hampered by the almost steady activation of the extensors of the thumb and of the abductor pollicis longus muscle (the muscle that pulls the thumb away from the other fingers in the plane of the palm). All the muscles involved in these actions are not innervated by the median nerve, even so, they seemed to lack their regular coordination. The carpo-metacarpal joint of the thumb, which usually allows a great variety of movements (a so-called saddle joint), was held forcefully in a position biased towards radial abduction. By pressing the proximal head of the first metacarpal bone towards the middle, I showed Hanoch that he could both stop that forceful abduction and start using the adductors. That was, at least passively, the first step towards the opposition of the thumb, and I then produced the movement simultaneously with flexion or extension of the wrist, and with pronation or supination of the forearm. Now Hanoch could start to aim the thumb towards the other fingers.

To enhance the function of the abductor pollicis brevis (the muscle that pulls the thumb away from the palm at a right angle to the palm's plane), I used the idea of the relative conjugate movement in the following manner: With Hanoch supine and his right forearm and palm flat on his chest and the thumb placed beneath the index finger, he was asked to lift his extended four fingers in the air together with the palm, leaving the thumb and also the forearm up to the wrist lying still on the chest. The *image* of that movement was quite easily translated into action, and upon realizing that the movement was in fact a changing of the angle between the thumb and the palm, that abduction was established.

During most of the time for weeks after that, Hanoch held a piece of rigid, lightweight plastic tube I had given him in his right hand (3 cm. in diameter, 20 cm. long, and with a rough surface). He held it with the ring finger and the little finger, both flexed, and tried to flex the other fingers over it, and to use any movement with it that he could already produce with the thumb (such as rolling the tube between thumb and index finger in various directions).

I also had him put his palm flat either on a table or somewhere on his face, fingers straightened out or slightly flexed, and make "scratching" movements with each finger tip longitudinally and transversally, without moving the other fingers; I also asked him to join the palms of both hands, with each finger touching its symmetrical opposite, and move the correspondent pairs of fingers in the plane of the palms and across that plane.

Some of the previous techniques are of importance to the method. It has already been mentioned that efficient monitoring of motor activity is dependent on afferent sensory feedback.

In any voluntary (goal-directed) activity, "negative" feedback makes it possible to evaluate any mismatch between an action already completed (or in the course of being performed) and its intended goal. This information causes the effectors to *diminish* that mismatch.

In Hanoch's case, almost all of the newly regained movements were monitored *visually* (the proprioceptive and touch sensations were still lacking). Without looking at his fingers and thumb he couldn't be sure if and how far the intended movement had been done. Now, by touching the palms and fingers of both hands, or interlacing the fingers of both hands, or touching his face with the fingers of his sensorily impaired hand, he added to his visual channel an alternative, substitutive sensory channel. The *skin* of his face or of his left hand "told" him about the movements of his right hand and fingers. The time had come to take up the flute.

The right thumb has a large role in fixing the flute's position by supporting it from below. The little finger is also involved in positioning the instrument, although most of the time it is pressing on one of the keys (it is required to do so by the fingering of most notes). With the forearm in pronation, the other three fingers descend from above on their respective keys, each of which also has an extra "trill key." These are little slender levers placed to the left, halfway between the principal circular keys.

Since Hanoch could not yet bring the thumb into full opposition and also could not flex the distal phalanges of the index and the middle fingers, he found that the middle phalanges of the three fingers were touching the keys instead of the finger tips. But he could reach all the keys (there was some difficulty with the index finger in the beginning), and we had only to close the holes in the centers of the three circular keys with pieces of cork. These holes are closed in normal playing by the respective finger tips as the keys are pressed down. That temporary device did not change the quality of the instrument in any appreciable amount.

Two serious difficulties had to be resolved immediately. First of all, when changing the fingering from one note to the next one, there are times when the first two or three fingers of the right hand have to press down (or to release) their keys *simultaneously;* otherwise an annoying intermediate tone is heard. Secondly, in situations in which the index finger had to hold down its key continuously for some time, it slid imperceptibly to the right and touched the nearby "trill key"—again producing an annoying, unwanted tone. Hanoch reacted to the second situation with a grimace of disgust. It was clear that the missing touch sensation prevented him from gaining control over that. I said to him, "Try not to be disturbed by these tones. They are, for the time being, the only source of information about how these fingers are behaving themselves on the flute. Take them as cues in knowing how to adjust and coordinate the movements of the fingers."

And so the *auditory sense* provided an alternative, substitutive channel of feedback for the motor functions of the fingers. That allowed him to proceed from the production of separate, discrete tones (staccato) to tied tones (legato).

I devised a number of exercises for Hanoch to do on the flute, so that he would learn to use less force with his affected fingers (he was doing this because of being unsure if the key was really being pressed down), and improve his agility by alternating easy fingerings back and forth with "difficult" ones. These exercises included dotted rhythms (using a given fingering for a very short while only), small groups of three or four short tones played very quickly in succession, fast scales (diatonic and chromatic) played in a saw-toothed fashion (four ascending notes, three descending, and so on), and others.

When, at the beginning of July, less than four months after the incident and two months after we started working, Hanoch spent more than an hour sight-reading all kinds of music (with someone accompanying him on the piano), he had the experience of realizing that in spite of all that had happened he was now on his way—he had just heard himself *making music.*

In the subsequent months, there was steady improvement.

The sensation of touch started to regenerate from proximal cutaneous innervations in the forearm, progressing distally at a slow pace; the distal phalanges of the fingers and thumb flexed; the *tips* of the fingers finally reached the keys on the flute easily; and Hanoch prepared for his reappearance on the concert stage. Besides all this, he was already writing, using a fork and knife, and driving his car.

When on March 20, 1979, approximately a year after the incident, Hanoch stepped on the stage of the overcrowded Jerusalem YMCA Auditorium for a concert of chamber music pieces by Bach, the public, knowing his story, gave him a standing ovation before the concert started. The music reviewer in *The Jerusalem Post* of March 22, 1979, declared:

> Tel-Oren showed a masterly skill, pitching his volume to enrich and not compete with the singer, yet never depriving his flute of positive individuality. . . . To hear a fine musician restored to his faculties after the terrible terrorist ordeal was an uplifting human and musical experience, and Hanoch Tel-Oren received a richly deserved, warm reception.

13. Improving the Ability to Perform*

There are a number of ways in which the physical or intellectual functions of a person can be considered impaired. There are those obvious cases requiring medical treatment, which can alleviate a given condition, cure it, or heal it. But quite separate from these are the many cases of otherwise "healthy" individuals who, when measured against certain standards of performance, are clearly functioning below their inherent capabilities.

Using a typical case history, I want to illustrate how the Feldenkrais method of Functional Integration may be of help in improving the overall quality of human functioning. This will also serve as an introduction to the theory and practice of the method.

I wish to focus specifically on the case of a person who had an obvious need to improve her performance of certain functions —as is often the case with athletes, musicians, actors, dancers, and other performers.

Most commonly, the way in which such persons will attempt to improve the level of performance is by trying harder, striving to do better, increasing one's effort, using "will power," or by repetitive exercises, all with the hope that the results will finally emerge during an actual performance or contest.

It is important to be aware of the philosophical assumptions underlying this common attitude, assumptions that are inherent in our Western culture and our educational practices. We

---

* First published in *Somatics*, vol. 1, no. 2 (1977).

hear the tutor saying, "Imitate a model, try hard, be serious, train both your will power and endurance, practice over and over again—otherwise you will fail." The underlying religious assumptions seem to be, "You are a sinner and will get your reward only the hard way; your ongoing punishment is for your entire life to be an unrelenting examination process demanding your constant self-sacrifice."

Despite the prevalence of this view, the result of such thinking is usually disappointing: very few persons ever succeed in improving their general abilities merely through repetitive striving. There are several reasons for this failure:

1. From the functional point of view, mere repetition involves going through, again and again, the same well-known pattern. Improvement, however, involves something quite different: a change in our patterns of functioning.

2. Conscious change of a pattern inevitably means learning: discerning and distinguishing between several possible patterns of movement or action, appreciating small differences and details, and being able to choose and act on these various possibilities.

3. To be able to discern minute differences in muscular patterns there must be a diminution in the overall proprioceptive sensory excitation—muscular effort must be cut to a minimum. This is in accordance with the well-known Weber-Fechner Law in physiology, which holds that the threshold of sensitivity to changes in sensory excitation is a certain fraction of the overall excitation already present.

For example, if I were holding a 20-pound weight in my hands, I might not perceive any change if someone added a half pound (one-fortieth) to what I was holding; but if I were holding only 10 pounds I could certainly perceive a weight change of half a pound. In the same way, the increased muscular tonus brought on by the effort of will power to repeat an action to the point of fatigue destroys the possibility of discerning small changes in muscular patterns, thus undermining the learning process.

4. The use of will power (effort) implies, psychologically, the juxtaposition of one's present level of performance against an ideal goal of performance not yet achieved. Obviously, the repetition of the same pattern means that subsequent repetitions promise little improvement. One is therefore frustrated, and this frustration, combined with a reinforced expectation of failure, may easily lead to a state of anxiety. The bodily component of the anxiety syndrome was first adequately described in *Body and Mature Behavior.* In essence, anxiety involves the inhibition of the extensor muscles and overactivation of the flexors. It is easy to imagine what this limited state of movement might mean for a long distance runner or for a concert pianist.

5. Neurologically, the repetition of a particular pattern of movement creates a well-trodden pathway along which efferent impulses may pass through the relevant synapses. This repetition diminishes the likelihood of alternative patterns arising; the one pattern becomes compulsive and so within the context of a certain activity there is no other possibility.

This analysis points to an obvious conclusion. If we intend to help someone in this predicament, the following must take place: the subject must be taught how to reduce the overall muscular tonus (perhaps mainly in the flexors), in order to be able to sense alternative patterns of movement. The subject can then choose the most appealing patterns, all the while understanding what is occurring. This gives the subject an increased awareness and learning ability with both reduced effort and greater efficiency.

But then, how can this be achieved? In order to describe, if only partially, the technical side of the Feldenkrais method and some of the thoughts underlying it, I will present the case of a pianist, describing the peculiar though not uncommon way she sat before her instrument and played, and the method of Functional Integration that allowed her to improve her general abilities of movement. The account outlines some of the manipulative procedures done during four half-hour sessions.

M. J., seventeen years old and a piano student at the conservatory, was already appearing in student concerts. She was urged by her teachers to work more on her finger agility, speed, and attack. During the preceding few months she had begun to have pain in her right wrist and forearm. It occurred when she was playing the piano and while writing. Even before this she had begun feeling discomfort and occasional pain in her neck, and she tended to get out of breath easily.

A physician who was consulted recommended that she cease playing the piano for the time being and try to get as much rest as possible. Upon learning this, her piano teacher suggested that she try the Feldenkrais method of Functional Integration.

Upon first seeing her, my initial impression was that the shoulders were drawn back and up, with very little head movement, and almost none in the torso; the sternum was depressed and the lower thoracic vertebrae and the corresponding ribs protruded backward. When in the sitting position her hip joints were flexed at an obtuse angle, so that the pelvis swayed backward. There was no lordosis in the lumbar region and the muscles of the abdomen were tight.

I checked first of all certain basic functions of the neuromotor system, three of which are worth particular mention:

1. The functions of the vertebral column. It was as if her vertebral column functioned like a nearly inflexible stick that connected the pelvis with the head. Because of this, her body movements were primarily those of moving the limbs relative to the torso; there was no movement that changed the distance and spatial relationship between shoulder girdle and pelvis.

The particular posture and movements associated with a personal pattern of motor functions constitute the self-image which one may have of oneself. In M. J.'s case it was something like the image of a cockroach. That image needed to metamorphose into a "cat image," so that she would understand and use the vertebral column as an elastically connected series of individual vertebrae that would not only allow but also demand participation of the movable parts of the torso and head during movements of the limbs.

In M. J.'s case, the torso was stiff because there was a simultaneous and continuous activation of both the extensors and flexors of the pelvis (the muscles of the back and abdomen). This was in sharp contrast to the normal and desirable reciprocal pattern of alternating use of antagonist muscles. This condition had come about without the subject being particularly aware of it.

I should mention again the fact that the activating of an agonist muscle has an inhibitory effect on the antagonist, and vice versa. The neural mechanism underlying these functions is extracortical, and may also be disturbed, as is shown by examples of hypertonicity or spasticity.

2. The functions of the shoulder blades. Not only were the shoulder blades almost motionless during movements of the arms, but the subject had only the vaguest notion of their location and their possibilities for movement. When I touched the lower tip of the right scapula, she said, "What's that hard bulge over my ribs there? Usually it's tender there, and sometimes it really hurts."

There were three pairs of antagonistic muscles, each showing an impairment of the action of their alternating reflex, as mentioned before: the muscles sliding the scapula up and down, those sliding inward and outward, and those rotating around the shoulder joint. The levator scapulae muscle was especially tense and also tender. Obviously, this state of affairs could not help but interfere with the free movement of the arms; because the range of movement was limited, she was automatically required to use more effort in her movements in order to overcome the resistance of those muscles binding the scapulae.

From a functional point of view the link between these two facts could be clearly observed in the nondifferentiated movements of the stiff torso, together with the shoulders and scapulae. The activation of the extensors of the back with the latissimus dorsi and serratus posterior muscles was simultaneous rather than synergetic: hence interfering. The possibility of differentiating the movements of these discrete muscles was just not a part of what Karl Pribram has termed "the image of achievement."

3. The functions of the rib cage. The basic patterns of movement that demand the participation of the ribs are those of bending and twisting the torso and of breathing. The bending and twisting movements of M. J.'s torso were inhibited and, since the big muscles around the ribs were constantly "holding" the torso, the ribs had little chance of participating in the action of breathing. The most striking detail was that the abdominal muscles, especially on the right side, were held tight, fixing the small ribs at a set distance from the pelvis.

Although the specific sequence of manipulations is too complex to describe here, the general procedures followed during these sessions illustrate two of the objectives of Functional Integration. The first objective is to teach the central nervous system to release the superfluous tonus of musculature of which the subject is unaware. This is done by the teacher taking over the effort made by these muscles.

For example, with the subject lying on the left side, the knees drawn up comfortably, I held her right elbow in a vertical position over the shoulder joint and, with my other hand, pushed the right scapula downward from beneath the armpit so that it could slide across the ribs in the direction of the vertebral column. By taking over the effort of the rhomboideus, serratus posterior, and latissimus dorsi muscles, I was able to obtain a response of "letting go." The antagonist muscles (serratus anterior and pectoralis) could then pull back, over the initial position of the scapula. It was then possible to lower the elbow to the side of the head easily, the lower tip of the scapula coming up smoothly with the movement.

This response originates in the motor cortex: The subject was aware of the change and gradually and with economy of effort, she began to perform the movement herself. After a few repetitions, she came to experience this as a conscious, deliberate pattern of movement, which meant that she had now learned to use her arm in a more functionally integrated manner.

I should also point out that during these manipulations the stretch reflex was evoked in the antagonist muscles, thus helping the scapula to move away from the spine.

A similar response was obtained with the subject lying on her stomach. I took over the work of the spinal extensors by bringing the insertions and origins nearer to one another. This was done on each side, respectively, by placing the palm of one of my hands over the pelvis and the other over the middle ribs where they bulged out slightly and where the extensors were tense and rope-like. In this position I pushed both hands toward one another, holding the ribs and pelvis in this proximal position.

After a while I began to feel resistance growing, which meant that the aided extensor muscles had ceased working, thus allowing the abdominal muscles to begin activating in opposition to this position. As soon as this response occurred, I let go and, unhampered by the overlying muscles of the back, the ribs suddenly rose and M. J. took a spontaneous, deep breath.

Then, with the subject lying on her back, I made use of the new freedom gained in the back muscles by lifting the shoulder girdle slightly (by pushing the scapulae up from beneath or by gently lifting the seventh cervical vertebra). In this way I was taking over some of the effort of the abdominal muscles by bringing origins and insertions nearer to one another. As soon as the abdominal muscles relaxed and ceased helping to lift the shoulders, I could feel the increased weight of the shoulders in my hands. At that moment the obvious happened: with the lower ribs now freed, M. J. again took a deep breath spontaneously. In this way the central nervous system acknowledges that a changed movement pattern is felt to be safe and comfortable.

The second objective of Functional Integration is to teach the central nervous system to use the skeletal structure as the main pathway for propagating the greater efforts, leaving the muscles free to direct the movements in the exact direction and degree needed. This means, for example, that in standing or sitting we should be able to rely on the skeleton to hold us upright, with only a minimum of muscular effort involved. In this way more musculature is available for voluntary movements.

When one pushes or strikes with the hand, the wrist, elbow, and even shoulder should be extended so that the work is performed by the large muscles of the torso. In this way, most of the force travels through the bones of the arms, which can easily support and transmit this force. Because it is weaker, the extensor of the elbow cannot efficiently bear and transmit the force, which should be shared by various muscles, in proportion to their strength.

In this instance the following manipulation was done: With the subject lying on the back, knees bent and feet planted on the table, I positioned the head so that I could gently push it downward in the direction of the pelvis. The direction of the pressure was through the vertebral column, so that at no time could there be a sensation of shearing (sliding at right angles to the direction of the pressure). The force of this manipulation travels primarily in a perpendicular direction through the facets of the vertebrae and, since the sole action of muscles is to contract, no muscular effort along the spine, conscious or unconscious, can prevent this perpendicular movement. By pushing the head in this manner and then beginning a rhythmical movement of pushing and releasing, I caused the work of the muscles of the torso to be taken over by the skeleton itself. According to the principle already mentioned, the torso muscles were released from their unconscious and unnecessary labors.

As soon as the subject's pelvis began rocking in response to the pressure, I let go of the head. Again, a deep breath occurred. When I placed her in a sitting position with the feet on the floor, she demonstrated the same alignment of her back: the head was high, the small of the back arched without any effort from the back muscles, the sternum rose easily with her breathing, the shoulders were wide and light—and she had a large smile on her face.

The results were these: M. J. now began to play the piano with increased efficiency and renewed self-confidence. The pain in her arm subsided completely, she felt no fatigue while playing, and her rate of progress was greater than before.

Conclusion: I have tried to show how one can be helped to become aware of the inhibitions imbedded in one's "image of achievement." These inhibitions and their dynamics can be described from the neuro-motor point of view, from the kinesthetic point of view of the subject (the immediate awareness of which movements are possible and which are impossible), and from a functional point of view. The functional line of thinking is instrumental in helping one to experience alternative patterns of organizing oneself, thus offering a freedom of choice and an enhanced ability to learn. This can come about by increasing one's awareness of what one is doing.

14. Remarks on Pain, Function, and Structure*

The number of people suffering from pain and disability caused by faulty functioning of the neuro-motor system is probably considerable. "Faulty functioning" means not only inefficiency in attaining a goal, but also a way of functioning *inadequate to the structure* of the executing parts. These executing parts include, of course, the central nervous system with its effective capability and adaptability, and the various parts of the body: bones, joints, muscles, in whatever state of health they may be. Parts of the immediate environment relevant to a particular activity should also be regarded as belonging to that structure when the question of inadequacy of functioning is being considered. Whenever muscular effort or expense of energy (energy in the purely physical sense) is not resulting in work being done, the only possible result will be wear and tear on joints, muscles, and ligaments, or damage by friction or contusion. Pain will often ensue, especially if that pattern is repeated.

Any inadequacy of the structure-function relationship can be effectively approached by way of the Feldenkrais method of Functional Integration *from the functional end* of the problem.

The question, "What's wrong with me there?" is, with the help of the Feldenkrais teacher, turned into, "What am I doing wrong there?" In other words, one's control over one's actions must be developed toward a higher, more differentiated, refined level, with increased adaptability and efficiency.

---

* First published in *Somatics*, vol. 3, no. 2 (1981).

A simple example is presented in the following case to illustrate this approach.

D. S., a woman of about fifty, was complaining of a sharp pain in the right knee. She couldn't bend the knee at more than a right angle and had difficulty in straightening it out when standing or walking. A thorough medical examination given to D. S. a few days earlier revealed, as she reported, no pathological findings in the knee region. Incidentally, D. S. showed me the X-ray pictures taken of both her knees. What puzzled me while looking at these X-rays was the peculiar position of the right fibula: in contrast to the left one, the head of the right fibula appeared, in the front view, to be shifted medially (towards the inside, behind the tibia), so that the overlapping parts of both the fibula and the tibia appeared significantly greater for the right knee than for the left one. In the lateral-view pictures, the head of the left fibula appeared to be aligned with the tibia, whereas the head of the right fibula "stuck out" backwards (over the tibia) about 7 mm.

Since the physician's examination had not yielded any findings—the implication being that there might be no *structural* deficiency—I presumed that it was D. S.'s way of *functioning* that needed improvement.

As an additional part of the picture, the right biceps femoris muscle (the outside hamstring) was taut and painfully sensitive to palpation. D. S. was amazed to find very soon that the tibialis posterior muscle was in a similar state: taut and painful to touch. This muscle, which has its lower part situated just behind the tibia on the inside of the leg, was used by D. S. synergistically with the biceps, which was characteristic of her distorted way of holding and moving the leg.

A few considerations should be mentioned concerning functions that involve the knee and the knee joint.

As for the movements in the knee joint besides the obvious flexing and extending of the knee, there is the rotation of the leg around its own axis (with the knee bent of course), the inward rotation done mainly with the popliteus muscle and the outward rotation done with the biceps femoris. The latter muscle, being attached to the head of the fibula, not only rotates both the tibia and the fibula in the knee joint but also slides the head of the fibula to the back of the tibia. The ligaments connecting these two bones usually allow this movement to a considerable extent. The forward sliding of the head of the fibula is done with the peroneal muscles, which have as their main function the eversion of the foot (the turning of the sole of the foot outward). As one of the hamstring muscles, the biceps femoris is involved in flexing the knee. This function gains preponderance with many people to such an extent that the rotation of the leg remains a rudimentary, undifferentiated, movement and, for some people, impossible to perform.

Dealing with the functions of the knee, one should not only examine movements in the joint, but also consider the role the knee has in the pupil's image of achievement in movements involving the change of the knee's location in space, such as the knee moving relative to the trunk (which means actually movement in the hip joint). For example, anyone experiencing pain in the knee will not wish his knee to be moved about, even without any movement in the knee joint (like left-right movements of the knee while sitting or lying on the back with the knees drawn up); instead, that person will stiffen around the hip joint. The teacher in Functional Integration might suggest that the person compensate for the difficulties in the knee joint by easy movements in the neighboring joints—the hip joint and the ankle joint—and then help to integrate these changes with motor functions involving other parts of the body. Such a compensation is likely to diminish the stress put on the knee joint, thus producing improvement.

Coming back to D. S., I shall describe part of the sequence of manipulations done in accordance with the principles of Functional Integration and with the foregoing analysis.

First lesson: By having D. S. lie on her stomach on a padded bench, with a soft support underneath her ankles, I produced the feeling of security in the knee—of not having to protect it against any "danger." Holding her toes, I gently flexed and extended the ankles, first the left one, then the right one. Nothing unexpected could happen to the "bad" leg, since the same movements had already been experienced in the "good" leg. Moreover, a comparison of the sensations in both legs was the first step towards an increased awareness of what was "there."

Gradually I began turning the heel right and left, until some rotation in the hip joint occurred, but with almost no movement in the knee joint. At each stage of the process I waited to sense whether D. S. experienced enough security (or perhaps curiosity?) to give up some of her defense patterns around the knee and elsewhere, and only then did I allow myself to go on and lead her into a further learning stage. With the tonus of some of her muscles lessened, I could then try to bend the knee slightly by lifting the ankle. I asked her to allow the extension easily, by letting the foot "fall down," even though I was supporting it. After she gained that little bit of control over the hamstrings (the biceps included), I rotated the leg, holding it flexed at the most comfortable angle, first without any change in the ankle joint and then combining the inward rotation with eversion of the foot—the very movement pattern she had avoided up until now.

To speed her awareness of the new pattern, I let her palpate her own biceps femoris (on the tendon, not far behind the knee joint), and asked her to resist my attempt to turn her heel to the outside (an inward rotation of the leg), or to let me rotate the leg and then to bring it back herself. Upon realizing that she was using *that* muscle for these actions, she actually constructed a new movement pattern out of its components: efferent (outgoing, motor) nerve impulses, afferent (incoming, sensory) nerve impulses, and a level of control that gave her the freedom of choice to do it or to stop it at will.

The same thing was then repeated with D. S. lying on the left side with the right knee drawn up at a right angle. This time, by rolling her right leg on the table to and fro, I could help her integrate that movement with the movement of the pelvis, after she allowed some relaxation of the hip joint and the lumbar spine.

Second lesson (two days later): I had D. S. lying on the table on her back, with the knees drawn up and the soles of the feet on the table, the legs slightly spread. The right foot appeared somewhat inverted (the sole of the foot turned to the inside), and the ankle shifted to the outside accordingly. I "helped" her exaggerate slightly this bias with two simultaneous maneuvers: with one hand I pushed the ankle from the inside outward to increase the inversion of the foot, while with my other hand I pushed the head of the fibula (by grasping the outer part of the leg, below the knee) towards the pelvis, in order to increase the outward rotation of the leg. Producing these as one movement had the effect of taking over some of the effort of both the biceps femoris and the tibialis posterior. After a few repetitions, the result was a lessening of the tonus of these muscles. Now, while still producing that movement, I shifted the emphasis gradually to the "coming back" phase and attempted to bring about the *eversion* of the foot until the entire sole was on the table and the ankle pushed slightly inward. I also attempted to make the *inward rotation* of the leg more complete by sliding the head of the fibula away from the pelvis. Suddenly D. S. could feel that her foot was securely planted on the table and that it was able to withhold downward pressure on the knee at right angles to the table without muscular effort, which means by relying on the bone structure.

It should be emphasized that a person's ability to align the bone structure so that it can take over the transmission of sizable forces (and the body weight) is always a prerequisite of efficient functioning. Such an alignment, when arrived at, is immediately recognized as comforting and beneficial, providing a feeling of power, but demanding no muscular exertion.

I also showed D. S. that, by having her leg in that inwardly rotated position, she could easily bend her knee to the limit, the heel touching the buttock, and she did so without any pain for the first time in months. Next came the extension of the knee, complete with the locking of the joint. With D. S. still on her back but now with the legs extended, I provided her with a sense of the skeleton's alignment by pushing slightly through the sole of the foot (first one, then the other) with the ankle slightly everted, and then releasing it, continuing this press-and-release movement until the pelvis, the chest, and finally the head were all rocking with the rhythm of my push. The breathing gradually became easier. Upon standing up, D. S. seemed to recognize that she was still in the same alignment she had experienced in the supine position. Now she walked about quite easily, as if she were gliding, apparently without any effort. The pain in the right knee was almost forgotten.

Two more lessons were given to consolidate the newly learned (or perhaps relearned) patterns of action, although they were hardly necessary.

The causal chain of occurrences leading to the sensation of pain is, in most cases, difficult to determine. In many instances, such an analysis seems impossible. This state of affairs is due to the fact that any one of these occurrences may be related to a large number of antecedent facts and may be a link in many pre-established sequences of behavior. To talk about "the cause of the pain" may, except in very obvious cases, be a gross over-simplification.

Nevertheless, in the case described here, one may safely assume that the head of the fibula, as it was held fixed in its displaced position, was impinging on the soft tissues encountered by it during the bending of the knee, thus producing irritation, inflammation, and pain. The other complaints also seemed to be of a predominantly functional character.

In the realm of structure and function, the practitioner of Functional Integration serves to help the pupil in learning to adjust and improve neuro-motor functioning. The body's structure and its immediate environment constitute the framework for that functioning, setting its limits or creating demands for its adjustment. Pain is often a signal of faulty functioning, and when that is the case, any approach applying itself only to the structural symptoms will have less chance of success.

15. Reflections on the Creative Process*

The psychological aspect of the creative process has always been a fascinating subject, and there have been a number of attempts to elucidate the mechanisms involved. Usually, creative processes are associated with artistic creativity, but often they are equally engaged in technological innovations or in mathematical creativity. The latter might include not only the invention and development of new branches of mathematics but also the field of problem-solving itself. Many people feel that this is a subject that can be taught. Indicative of this is the fact that *heuristics* is presently undergoing a revival—as witness the excellent book by G. Polya, *How to Solve It.***

All these processes and many more that occur in everyday life can be properly included under the heading of "creative processes," even if this means stretching the usual and somewhat constricted connotation of that term slightly. They have as a common factor the inventiveness of the person who is active in the process—the "creator"—who has the ability of creating a new, perhaps unique, pattern of conduct; of maximizing a situation; of expressing a thought or a feeling in a unique way; or of making new combinations of materials and using the process as a way of answering a particular question in a corresponding field of action.

There is always some way of evaluating the outcome of such

---

* First published in *Somatics*, vol. 1, no. 4 (1978).
** (Princeton: Princeton University Press, 1971).

a process. This evaluation can be done not only by someone outside the process of creation, but it can also be done by the "creator" *during* the process of creation. If we can show, in this latter instance, how such an evaluation is done and by what criteria, then we may well have taken a large stride toward understanding that most elusive of processes: the process of creation.

As a contribution to this field, I want to explore certain processes in the Feldenkrais method of Functional Integration that seem to be "creative" in this broader sense. The reason for choosing Functional Integration is that, during the process of doing it, the teacher is very conscious of his or her activity, because the objective of this method is, insofar as possible, to convey to the subject information concerning his or her patterns of neuro-motor organization. A second reason is that, at its best, Functional Integration involves the heuristic challenge of searching for the most efficient patterns of movement for each individual. This is a procedure moving in a direction counter to any mechanical or standardized technique.

To begin, I will give a very brief description of Functional Integration, and then as I develop my point, some of the illustrations given will show the interesting ways in which this method operates.

Functional Integration might be defined as a technique of body manipulation by which the teacher gives the subject an awareness of the neuro-motor system in terms of the fixed set of movement patterns that are habitually used and habitually avoided, thus providing the experience of new, alternative movement patterns that may be assimilated. As "material," the teacher has the subject's body and the typical ways the subject has of using it, namely, the particular ways in which the subject's central nervous system is "wired in" in respect to the motor system and the way it reacts to stimuli. To communicate with the central nervous system, the teacher uses both his and the subject's sensory channels, such as touch and vision, but primarily the kinesthetic channel, through which we sense body position, movement, and muscular effort. Since almost no words are spoken in Functional Integration, the "words" of this nonverbal language-communication are the images of movement patterns.

I will limit the discussion of the realm of these "images" by not going into a neuro-physiological description of the processes involved. In fact, a neuro-physiological description of the processes involved in Functional Integration has not yet been attempted. This is closely linked with the paucity of research, on the neuronal level, of the imagining and learning processes in general, although some significant steps have been taken in researching the latter topic.

Functional Integration is most useful and needed in the cases of persons having problems of neuro-motor coordination, whatever the cause, or who need some improvement in their efficiency of functioning.

"We act and move according to our self-image." This is the central idea in Moshe Feldenkrais's *Awareness Through Movement*. Confining ourselves to neuro-motor functioning, this means that there is a set of movement patterns that a person is typically bound to perform and to conceive of himself performing. In addition to this, there may exist certain defense mechanisms which, at a less-than-conscious level, prevent this person from performing movement patterns different from the typical set. This is to say that there are neuro-motor safeguards or anti-patterns which defend against the performance of certain actions—"That's not me!" "I can't do a thing like that!" "I'm too old, too grown up, too cultured, serious, weak, slow, stiff, to do that!"

The following would be an illustration of this point: Take the case of a person who, when arising from a sitting position, does so without straightening up fully, and so stands bent slightly forward, with a round back, a sunken chest, and a slight bend in the hip joints. If this is the characteristic posture, it is extremely difficult to convince one *with words* that one is really much taller than it appears. One is normally unaware that the muscles of the abdomen are tense and shortened and that, most likely, other flexor muscles such as the flexors of the thighs and the sterno-cleido-mastoidei are tense as well. To complete the picture, the extensor muscles of the back are bearing the weight of the body, preventing it from collapsing altogether, and thus engaging most of the body's large muscles in the act of holding the posture, which makes it impossible for other muscles to perform useful movements at the same time. More often than not, such a person will complain of tiredness, backache, weak legs, shortness of breath, and, in general, low vitality.

In what way does a set of movement patterns such as this achieve dominance in the body? Some movement patterns are obviously hereditary: they are philogenetically "wired into" the central nervous system (such as swallowing, breathing, sucking). Other patterns are consciously and freely chosen; many persons have the belief that the majority of their movement patterns have been deliberately chosen. But there is a third way in which these patterns are adopted. There are learned patterns that are ontogenetically wired in through education, imitation, habit, or compulsion—patterns that are acted out more or less automatically. By "compulsion" I mean not only compulsion from the outside world, but also from the way we react to discomfort, stress, or pain; by instinctively contracting certain muscles *as a defense mechanism,* which through repetition becomes habit-forming.

If one is to influence and, perhaps, change the fixed set of a subject's movement patterns, one must normally deal with two different situations. (1) First of all, we encounter the situation in which some previously used—and perhaps quite efficient—patterns have become inhibited for a number of reasons of which the subject is unaware. Very often this is an instance of what Feldenkrais has termed "the body pattern of anxiety." In this case, the teacher must help reinstate the previously used patterns, unless there are obvious physiological reasons preventing it, such as injury or trauma. The subject is helped to recognize these patterns as feasible, beneficial, and enriching—typically, this is the "Oh, yes!" experience. (2) In the second situation, one must teach the subject new patterns of movement that were previously nonexistent or were functionally lost after central or peripheral lesions. In this instance, the subject does not relearn an old pattern, but learns and discovers something new about the body and its possibilities: this is the "Aha!" experience.

In either case, the practical way of proceeding is the same, because one must take advantage of the same learning capacity of the subject's central nervous system.

Let us continue with the case described above, in which a person has overactivated flexors and inhibited extensors. The teacher might ask this person to lie down on the left side, with the knees drawn up comfortably, and with a soft support beneath the head. Comfort is one of the essential conditions; it enables the subject to discern and differentiate minute changes in movement patterns that will be nonverbally "proposed" by the teacher.

The *first step* could be to increase this sense of comfort by helping the hardworking flexors of the abdomen in their effort. The teacher might do this by slightly pushing the subject's pelvis in a diagonal direction (from behind) so as to shorten the right abdominal muscles, the effect of which is to release these muscles and allow the pelvis to come back easily, perhaps beyond the initial position. Or the teacher might push the chest diagonally (from behind) to achieve the same effect as above. The teacher could also produce both of the above movements simultaneously to achieve the same effect, or could push the shoulder (or the spinal column near the shoulder) from above the collar bone toward the pelvis, releasing it rhythmically until the pelvis begins rocking with the same rhythm. There are still other options: The teacher could sit behind the subject, holding the small ribs of the right side in place with one hand and gently pushing the pelvis forward with the other hand; or, the same as above, but pressing the shoulder blade forward rather than the ribs. All of these manipulations can result in a lessening of the muscular tonus of the abdomen, provided that they impart *a feeling of security* to the subject—namely, a feeling that the manipulations are helpful and do not threaten the habitual movement-patterns directly.

Which of these many possibilities should be used by the teacher and in what order? One might think that this could be left to trial and error, but, unfortunately, such fumbling would leave the subject feeling insecure or even annoyed. The experienced teacher, on the basis of the initial palpations and visual observations, selects the movements that will work. However this may vary from subject to subject, that which "works" is that which changes rigidity to flexibility, from holding the breath to engaging the ribs easily in breathing, and from resisting new movement to allowing and preferring it. Constant checking and confirmation of what works and what does not work must go on throughout the session.

The lessening of tonus in the abdominal muscles also increases the possibility of improving the quality of other functions, such as twisting the torso, arching the small of the back, and breathing with the participation of the ribs—all of these having been hampered by the previously contracted abdominal muscles. These new movements are a further enhancement and consolidation of the change that has already taken place, integrating this change into more patterns of movement.

The *next stage* of work will be the following: With the person in the same position as before, the teacher applies pressure in a forward direction from behind the pelvis and the right-side ribs toward a mutual convergence or, inversely, arches the small of the back into a divergence of the pelvis and chest. Or, the teacher presses the pelvis at the right hip joint, down and back, extending the right arm horizontally up and forward. Or the teacher may execute both of these movements alternately (rocking) or simultaneously (twisting the spine); extending the head slightly in the direction of the spine and then releasing (so that the pelvis rocks). There are still other possibilities.

Here again, as to the choice of manipulations and their sequence, the same can be said as before: *the teacher is continuously aware of the response of the subject's system and is adapting his actions to the reactions of the subject.*

In some cases one can proceed to a *third stage*—a summing up of the experience that the subject has just had. Feldenkrais refers to this third stage operation as a *clé de voûte* or "keystone." In this particular case, the manipulations might consist of the following: With the subject in the same position as before, the teacher supports—from below—the vertebra (or group of vertebrae) nearest the supporting horizontal plane, so that (1) the arch in the small of the back is slightly increased, (2) the lateral curve downward of the spine (caused by the subject's position) is slightly straightened out, and (3) the distance between the right-side small ribs and the pelvic bone is increased. Thus, by having support of the spine provided, the subject can feel the "proposed" new spatial orientation of the body, an orientation that enhances and facilitates a number of movement-patterns. The subject may then become aware that what is "proposed" may, in principle, be only a minute change in posture, but it is a change that bears directly on a variety of vital functions.

Let us now return to the definition of the "creative process" proposed earlier. We can see that the work of Functional Integration occurs as a continuous, creative series of evaluative responses to the sensory feedback perceived by the teacher-creator. The work is constantly monitored: "Is that too much for the subject?" "Will *that*, perhaps, please the subject?" "Has the subject understood what is being done?" "Does it work or doesn't it?" In brief, the proof of a new pattern is in its working. The outcome of the process may be considered to be *an answer to a question or a problem concerning the subject.* This answer may not, at the beginning, be something that the teacher is fully aware of, but this awareness emerges as the ultimate outcome of the procedure.

I believe that the same situation occurs in other creative processes: in the attitude of the "creator" toward the "material," in the nature of the activity, and in the procedure of continuously checking the outcome throughout the process. The outcome of the process is experienced by the creator as giving an answer to a question or problem. In some instances, a question may be proposed uniquely for the purpose of having it answered, as is the case, consciously or unconsciously, with most creations of art.

Bibliography

Bateson, Gregory. *Steps to an Ecology of Mind.* New York: Ballantine, 1975.

Cailliet, Rene, M.D. *Scoliosis, Diagnosis and Management.* Philadelphia: F. A. Davis, 1975.

Hanna, Thomas. *The Body of Life.* New York: Knopf, 1980.

Feldenkrais, Moshe. *Adventures in the Jungle of the Brain: The Case of Nora.* New York: Harper & Row, 1977.

Feldenkrais, Moshe. *Awareness through Movement.* New York: Harper & Row, 1972.

Feldenkrais, Moshe. *Body and Mature Behavior.* London: Routledge and Kegan Paul, 1949; New York: International Universities Press, 1950; New York: International Universities Press, paperback, 1970.

Feldenkrais, Moshe. *The Elusive Obvious.* Cupertino, California: Meta Publications, 1981.

Scientific American, September 1979.